Louise Baxiot

D0519497

Contents

Foreword

In the five years since the last edition of *The Minor Illness Manual* was published, we have witnessed significant change in the healthcare delivery systems within our NHS. Primary care has always, quite literally, been at the forefront of provision, but today we see an ever more significant emphasis on care and treatment of people close to their home, or indeed workplace.

As our hospitals rightly become the centres of technical excellence required to treat the very sick and critically injured, we have developed primary care solutions to healthcare needs which were considered radical and innovatory when the authors compiled their first edition. Minor illness care has expanded beyond the GP surgery to a range of other facilities, including the NHS Walk-in Centres, many of which are exclusively staffed by nurses. Community pharmacists are also expanding their role in first contact care.

The Minor Illness Manual is an excellent resource to all of those who need an easily accessible summary of common complaints and presentations accompanied by concise care and treatment guidelines. An essential tool for today's primary care practitioner.

Mark Jones
Chief Nurse Adviser, Ministry of Health
Wellington, New Zealand
Previously, Director, UK Community Practitioners' and
Health Visitors' Association
September 2005

Preface to third edition

Since the first edition of this book was published in 1997, there has been a major shift in the expectations of both patients and health professionals about the management of acute illness. The idea that a specially trained nurse could advise safely on a wide range of symptoms has changed from being revolutionary, to being acceptable, to being expected. Financial pressure on the National Health Service has caused managers to actively promote nurse-led services for out-of-hours primary care cover. As a consequence, many patients with minor illness have benefited from the rapid access, holistic approach and advice on self-management which a specialist nurse can provide. But this is not a cheaper option; research shows that such nurses spend longer with patients than doctors, creating high levels of patient satisfaction but no reduction in the cost per consultation.

Minor illness is only minor in retrospect. In making a clinical assessment it is often impossible to exclude serious disease, and only possible to judge that it is very unlikely. Increasing fear of litigation and complaint has made general practitioners more cautious, but they remain more comfortable than nurses with accepting the personal responsibility which such decisions entail. This is not just a consequence of their different career paths; most nurses' salaries are not yet adequate recompense for carrying such a burden of uncertainty. Ideally, concerns about the increasing referral of patients with acute illness into secondary care can best be addressed by arrangements which permit 'First Contact' nurses to seek advice from experienced general practitioners.

The medicalisation of our society continues unabated, with polypharmacy flourishing on a scale which would have been impossible to envisage in the days when all prescriptions had to be written by hand. Nurses may find that their previous training has not prepared them for a world in which they frequently need to identify drug/drug and drug/illness interactions, nor for patients who are eager to identify almost any symptom as a side effect of their medicines (inevitably identified somewhere within the small print of their Patient Information Leaflets). It is crucial that nurses who manage minor illness consolidate their knowledge of pharmacology, even if they are not personally responsible for issuing prescriptions. The nurse prescribing programme continues to expand, testing the boundaries between nursing and medicine. An Extended Formulary Nurse Prescriber qualification will enhance the autonomy of nurses who specialise in the management of minor illness, but it is not a qualification in clinical assessment and cannot, on its own, provide them with sufficient clinical experience and diagnostic skills to practise safely in this role.

Change can be viewed as exciting or challenging. Around the United Kingdom nurses in general practice, Walk-in Centres and Minor Injuries Units are adapting to changing roles. Many find great satisfaction in developing their career in ways which encourage the critical analysis of evidence, reflection on experience and expanding clinical judgement.

Gina Johnson
Ian Hill-Smith
Chris Ellis
September 2005

About the authors

Stopsley Group Practice
All of the authors of this book work together in a Royal College of General Practitioners (RCGP) accredited research practice near Luton Airport which cares for around 6000 patients. In 1996 this practice developed an innovative educational programme for nurses on the management of minor illness. By mid-2005, 610 nurses had attended their seminar weeks, and over 400 had completed six-month clinical placements and achieved university accreditation.

Dr Gina Johnson graduated from Guy's Hospital in 1979, and has worked as a general practitioner since 1983, being actively involved in primary care research from the beginning. She is very aware of the limitations of Western medicine, which led her to study for an MSc in medical anthropology. She has been a T'ai Chi practitioner since 1999, and has recently started to use acupuncture in the surgery in an attempt to reduce her dependence on the prescription pad.

Dr Ian Hill-Smith started publishing research papers while studying for his first degree in anatomy before graduating in medicine from University College Hospital, London, in 1980. Despite the distractions of becoming a member of the Royal Colleges of both Physicians and General Practitioners, and an MD on drugs prescribed in primary care, he remains fascinated by fundamental science and loves the freedom only a generalist can feel.

Dr Chris Ellis graduated from the Royal Free Hospital in 1982. He has been a general practitioner for the best part of 20 years, and still enjoys the variety and challenges that it brings. Chris is the rock on which the practice stands. His hard-working dedication to everyday primary care allows the others to pursue their (sometimes wild) ideas. *(We wrote this bit for him because he is too modest!)*

Amber Kelly moved from health visiting to practice nursing with Stopsley Group Practice, and then gained qualifications in family planning, diabetes nursing, and teaching, and a degree in community nursing. She trained as an extended formulary nurse prescriber while completing minor illness training, and is currently involved in nursing research. Her greatest personal growth came from attaining a degree in literature and historical studies and on achieving a master's degree in literature.

Rhona Rollings has been a practice nurse for nearly 20 years. She was a pioneer in the development of minor illness specialist education, and has been involved with the course since its inception, as a lecturer and mentor to the students on six-month clinical placements. She has qualifications in family planning and asthma, is an extended formulary nurse prescriber and community practice teacher, and has just completed a degree in healthcare.

Acknowledgements

We would like to thank our staff at the Stopsley Group Practice for their ongoing support, especially Lorraine Dakin, without whose skills and patience the Minor Illness Course would never have been possible. We are grateful to the many nurses who have attended our courses and seminars, who have taught us so much.

David Johnson, Medical Librarian at the Luton and Dunstable Hospital, provided invaluable help with researching the evidence.

We also thank our patients, for allowing us to learn from their experiences of minor illness.

The nurse's perspective on changes and safe practice in primary care

The delivery of care in the NHS, particularly with respect to primary care, has changed rapidly over the past few years and since the publication of the last edition of *The Minor Illness Manual*. Government initiatives and their implementations have seen nurses move forward at an almost unprecedented rate, and what was once viewed as innovative practice, albeit sceptically by some, has rapidly become the norm.[1,2] Walk-in centres, NHS Direct, out-of-hours services, nurse consultants and the advent of community matrons are just some instances where nurse-led care is evident and thriving, and new roles are being created. Career pathways, which were once limited, have now developed in the primary care setting.

Such progress has been needs based. In response to growing consumerism, primary care trusts (PCTs) are obliged to offer patients an appointment with a primary healthcare professional within 24 h and a general practitioner (GP) within 48 h. This, together with the sheer volume of people presenting and requesting same-day appointments, the decline in the number of doctors, and the shift of care from the secondary to primary care setting, have all contributed to the emergence of higher levels of practice among primary care nurses. Public confidence in nurses as the first point of contact has grown, and nurses have proved themselves capable of extending their roles, scope of practice and competence in the management of conditions that were once the domain of the medical profession. In order to enhance these roles, a change in law to allow independent extended and supplementary nurse prescribing was passed. The Health and Social Care Act (2001) permitted the inclusion of a further group of independent nurse prescribers, allowing those previously excluded to prescribe, once trained, from the Nurse Prescribers' Extended Formulary (NPEF).[3] The NPEF includes all general sales list (GSL) items (those not requiring a pharmacist's supervision), all pharmacy (P) medicines (those requiring a pharmacist's supervision), and a number of specific prescription-only medicines (POMs) including contraceptives, vaccinations and some antibiotics. This was to enable all nurses working within roles that have this need and opportunity, to prescribe from the extended nurse formulary.[4] A consultation on future options for the NPEF and the development of nurse prescribing is currently under way.[5] Historically, independent prescribing is one of the biggest changes to happen to the nursing profession and should prove invaluable in the management of minor illness and the attainment of autonomy, while benefiting patients through quicker access to treatment and continuity of care. There are now more than 3800 nurses registered as extended formulary nurse prescribers (EFNPs),[6] still a long way from the government's ideal of 10 000 by 2004. Although the NPEF is often perceived as limited and a reason to not undertake training, as the formulary in *The Minor Illness Manual* demonstrates, the majority of minor ailments seen in primary care and the drugs available for their treatment are covered. In a role where the nurse is already assessing the patient and recommending the necessary treatment it would seem logical for the nurse to legitimise her own 'prescribing' rather than expect the GP to accept the responsibility. To simplify the complicated process of cross-referencing drugs and their conditions for treatment with the *British National Formulary (BNF)*, and to minimise this need, the medicines available for EFNPs have been highlighted in the formulary in *The Minor Illness Manual*. The most obvious shortfall is for treatment of upper respiratory tract infections where a nurse may assess, diagnose, recommend antimicrobials, and generate a prescription which must then be signed by a doctor. However, prior to extended prescribing, all prescriptions generated by nurses in general practice required a doctor's signature, except those prescribed under the limited original Nurse Prescribers' Formulary for District Nurses and Health Visitors. Retrospectively, although prescribing hasn't moved as far as some would wish, it has advanced considerably.

In England, the course for extended formulary and supplementary nurse prescribers is delivered by institutes of higher education at no less than first degree level with at least 26 taught days and 12 days learning in practice with a medical supervisor.[7] Approved by the Nursing and Midwifery Council (NMC), nurses who successfully complete the training programme have their qualifications recorded on the NMC register. For the management of minor illnesses, modules are available similar to the type delivered nationally by Stopsley Group Practice. This level 3 module is validated at 45 Credit Accumulation and Transfer Scheme (CATS) points, while other similar minor illness management modules, depending on validation by the institutes concerned, attract differing CATS points at level 3. For those nurses unable to access taught programmes, an uncredited distance learning pack is available in conjunction with, as all modules are, supervision in practice.[8] The nurse practitioner degree programme, run by the Royal College of Nursing (RCN), comprises six level 3 modules with supervision and support from medical and nursing facilitators, and results in a BSc(Hons) Nurse Practitioner (primary health care) qualification. This programme has been franchised, and is delivered by some universities via distance learning and by some at postgraduate level. More recently a postgraduate programme in First Contact Care has been developed. The MSc for First Contact practitioners is managed by the NHS University and delivered in association with Sheffield Hallam University, taking a minimum of 18 months to complete. Such diversity in educational packages has been accompanied by confusion and profusion in the titles used by nurses practising at higher levels. The roles of clinical nurse specialists, developed to enable nurses to take on work that was once the responsibility of doctors, often reflect disparity in terms of experience, expertise and competence. Many nurses who have successfully completed undergraduate modules for the management of minor illnesses have taken on the title of nurse practitioner without completing the necessary degree pathway. While nurse titles remain unrecorded on the NMC register, it raises, in an age of increasing consumerism, the question of quality assurance.[9] In order to address present disparities and set a standard that the public can expect from nurses working at higher levels of practice, the NMC is proposing to establish a regulated level of practice beyond registration. Currently out for consultation is a framework for a standard of expected proficiency and a requirement for further registration, proposing the creation of an additional sub-part of the nursing register for advanced nurses.[10]

All nurses are familiar with the concept of legal and professional accountability. Accountability for practice, knowledge and competence lies ultimately with the registered nurse as embedded in the NMC Code of Professional Conduct:[11]

- You must keep your knowledge and skills up-to-date throughout your working life. In particular, you should take part regularly in learning activities that develop your competence and performance. (6.1)

- To practise competently, you must possess the knowledge, skills and abilities required for lawful, safe and effective practice without direct supervision. You must acknowledge the limits of your professional competence and only undertake practice and accept responsibilities for those activities in which you are competent. (6.2)

- If an aspect of practice is beyond your level of competence or outside your area of registration, you must obtain help and supervision from a competent practitioner until you and your employer consider that you have required the requisite skill and knowledge. (6.3)

- You have a responsibility to deliver care based on current evidence, best practice and, where applicable, validated research when it is available. (6.5)[11]

Appropriate professional indemnity insurance is essential. In addition to the indemnity provided by professional bodies, for nurses working in general practice, the Medical Defence Union and The Medical Protection Society have group schemes to cover both the GPs and the practice nurses employed by them. It is advisable to provide these bodies with copies of job descriptions for nurses who manage minor illness in general practice. Job descriptions should be up-to-date, comprehensive and accurately reflect all aspects of the role being undertaken. This is particularly pertinent with the new NHS pay and career structure, the Agenda for Change (AfC), which gives nurses the opportunity to move away from dated clinical grading and Whitley scales to a pay system that links job evaluations with the knowledge and skills necessary to fulfil them and to the responsibilities involved. Although not currently extended to nurses employed in general practice, the RCN strongly believes that AfC rates of pay should include all nurses employed by GPs;[12] and best practice and financial rewards within the General Medical Service (GMS) contract are linked to its implementation.[13]

Continuing professional development and clinical supervision are integral to safe and effective practice. Informal networks to provide support and supervision are essential for nurses in general practice experiencing difficulty accessing clinical supervision. Such networks act, in the absence of formal clinical supervision, similarly, by developing and extending support, knowledge, skills and understanding, while monitoring quality of care. Here in Luton we have developed our own nurse prescribers' group, formalised at its establishment by a set of terms of reference and the involvement of a PCT pharmacist. It is open to all nurses who are qualified as EFNPs, and the group meets regularly, feeding back to the PCT Nurse Prescribing Steering Group as appropriate. Protected time for such meetings is necessary and should be negotiated with employers. It is important for employers to recognise the value of this support in order to reduce the stress and insecurities that can often accompany higher levels of practice. As more non-medical prescribing leads come into post, opportunities to formalise this type of peer support through the implementation of clinical supervision should improve. Continuing professional development is also inherent in professional responsibility and clinical governance, and is paramount to the delivery of care and as evidence of competence to practise.

Once underpinned by education and training, *The Minor Illness Manual* offers nurses guidelines to support decision making for the treatment of illness commonly presenting in primary care. In individual GP practices, these guidelines should be agreed jointly by doctors and the minor illness nurses. If discrepancies arise, possibly where there are local variations in antimicrobial treatment or disagreement regarding treatment, new guidelines pertinent to that practice should be written and documented. The guidelines can be used as protocols which are followed to enable safe and effective practice. For nurses working in primary care settings other than GP practices, patient group directions (PGDs) may be used for the supply or administration of medicines. This is not regarded as a form of prescribing and, therefore, no specific training is required in order to supply medicines in this way.

Ongoing changes in primary care mean opportunities for nurses have never been better; and nurses are continuing to be encouraged to adopt higher levels of practice for the delivery of *The NHS Plan*.[1] When the first edition of *The Minor Illness Manual* was published in 1997, the emergence of a minor illness nurse appeared radical. This role, and that of nurse practitioners, are now central components of general practice and essential to the delivery of primary care today.

References

1 Department of Health (2000) *The NHS Plan*. The Stationery Office, London.
2 Department of Health (2001) *Liberating the Talents: helping PCTs and nurses deliver the NHS Plan*. The Stationery Office, London.
3 *Health and Social Care Act* (2001). The Stationery Office, London.
4 Department of Health (2004) *Extending Independent Nurse Prescribing within the NHS in England. A guide for implementation* (2e). www.dh.gov.uk (accessed 8 June 2005).
5 Medicines and Healthcare products Regulatory Agency (2005) *Consultation on Options for the Future of Independent Prescribing by Extended Formulary Nurse Prescribers*. www.dh.gov.uk/assetRoot/04/10/40/58/04104058.pdf
6 News Round-Up (2005). www.nurse-prescriber.co.uk/news/News
7 Department of Health (2004) *Extended Independent Nurse Prescribing Within the NHS in England. A guide for implementation* (2e). www.dh.gov.uk (accessed 8 June 2005).
8 Johnson G, Hill-Smith I and Ellis C (2000) *Minor Illness. An open learning programme for nurse-led clinics in primary care*. Radcliffe Medical Press, Oxford.
9 Kelly A (2004) What's in a name? One practice nurse's perspective. *Community Pract* **77**: 224–6.
10 Nursing and Midwifery Council. Consultation on a framework for the standard of post-registration nursing. www.nmc-uk.org (accessed 8 June 2005).
11 Nursing and Midwifery Council (2002) *Code of Professional Conduct*. Nursing and Midwifery Council, London.
12 Royal College of Nursing (2004) *Nurses employed by GPs. RCN guidance on good employment practice*. Royal College of Nursing, London.
13 Royal College of Nursing (2005) *Agenda for Change. A guide to the new pay, terms and conditions in the NHS*. Royal College of Nursing, London.

Introduction

General advice

History
- listening is the greatest skill. What is the patient's agenda?
- open questions may reveal hidden concerns
- most diagnoses are made on the history – 'listen to the patient: he is telling you the diagnosis'

Examination
- this may reveal important signs, but will also serve to reassure the patient

Tests
- only useful if the management depends on the result
- may give false-positive results and cause unnecessary concern

Action
- discuss the options and agree the proposed plan of management with the patient
- ask the patient to contact the most appropriate NHS service if:
  - the situation worsens
  - there is no improvement within a specified time

Caution
- although guidelines support clinical judgement, they can never replace experience and intuition

Immunocompromised patients need special care, and will probably require antibiotic therapy, even for minor infections.

By immunocompromised, we mean:

- patients on immunosuppressant drugs, e.g. prednisolone, azathioprine, methotrexate, ciclosporin, chemotherapy
- patients with medical conditions which reduce their immune response, e.g. HIV, leukaemia, diabetes, post-splenectomy, malnutrition.

It is crucial that you identify these patients by taking a careful history.

Upper respiratory tract

Sore throat

History
- duration
- fever/malaise
- recurrent problems
- immunocompromised
- on medication which may cause agranulocytosis, e.g. carbimazole, mirtazapine

Examination
- examine throat – asking the patient to yawn or pant may improve the view. Consider using a tongue depressor if the back of throat is not visible (but beware of epiglottitis, *see* below)
- assess inflammation of pharynx
- look for exudates on tonsils
- check neck for enlarged lymph nodes (cervical lymphadenopathy)
- look for a macular rash (small red patches, not raised)

Tests
- full blood count (FBC) and Paul Bunnell test may be helpful to diagnose glandular fever, if symptoms persist for longer than a week
- urgent FBC should be requested if patient on drugs causing agranulocytosis

Action
- antibiotics are of marginal benefit in most cases, and at best will only shorten the illness by 24 h. Against this must be weighed the cost to the patient (prescription charge, risk of side-effects) and to society (antibiotic resistance, medicalisation of illness). Give antibiotics if immunocompromised, or if severe malaise or macular rash (scarlatina) present

- in a teenager these symptoms and signs are more likely to be due to glandular fever, so antibiotics should generally be avoided unless there is severe malaise. Do not use amoxicillin for sore throat in this age group; this may cause a rash in a patient with glandular fever (the rash is disease specific, not due to an allergy). Consider tests above

Prescription/ over-the-counter drugs (OTC)

- symptomatic treatment for most patients (ibuprofen or paracetamol, benzydamine spray)

- if an antibiotic is indicated in adults and children aged 10 years and over, give penicillin V for 10 days

- if an antibiotic is indicated in children under 10 years, we recommend amoxicillin suspension for 7 days. Although it is more likely to cause side-effects than penicillin V, in our experience young children find the taste of penicillin V suspension unpleasant and often refuse to take it

- if allergic to penicillin, use erythromycin, or clarithromycin if erythromycin not tolerated

Refer to doctor

- immediately if:

  - child very sick, drooling, cannot swallow (possible *epiglottitis*, do not examine throat)

- urgently if:

  - large swelling around one tonsil (possible *quinsy*, may need surgery)

  - on drugs that can cause agranulocytosis. If this is suspected, take immediate advice from a doctor regarding stopping the medication

References

- Del Mar C, Glasziou P and Spinks AB (2004) Antibiotics for the symptoms and complications of sore throat (Cochrane Review). *The Cochrane Library, Issue 2, 2004.* Update Software, Oxford.
- Little P, Williamson I, Warner G *et al.* (1997) Open randomised trial of prescribing strategies in managing sore throat. *BMJ* **314**: 722–7.
- Wethington JF (1985) Double-blind study of benzydamine hydrochloride, a new treatment for sore throat. *Clin Ther* **7**: 641–6.

'Swollen glands' (enlarged cervical lymph nodes)

History	• sore throat
	• fever
	• duration of swelling
Examination	• number and size of enlarged nodes
	• throat
Test	• FBC and Paul Bunnell if symptoms last more than a week in a teenager or young adult
Action	• explain that the 'glands' are the body's defence against infection
Prescription/OTC	• ibuprofen or paracetamol if pain is severe
Refer to doctor	• if there is a single very large painful node (may contain an abscess)
	• if lymph nodes are hard or enlarging progressively over two weeks or more (may be a sign of lymphoma, leukaemia or tuberculosis)

Mumps

This was previously a disease of children which had become very rare following the introduction of mumps vaccination. Most cases are without serious consequence, but complications include orchitis, pancreatitis, viral meningitis and risk of miscarriage between 12 and 16 weeks' gestation. In 2004, as a consequence of the measles mumps and rubella vaccination (MMR) scare, there was a large increase in mumps cases in the 16 to 25 age group. These people were born too late to have received two doses of mumps vaccine, and too early to have been exposed to the wild virus.

History	• swelling/pain of parotid glands (in front of the ears)

- dry mouth, worse on swallowing or chewing
- fever
- malaise
- headache
- drowsiness/photophobia/vomiting
- abdominal or testicular pain
- in women, check for possible pregnancy

Examination
- parotid glands (swelling may be unilateral or bilateral)

Tests
- confirmation of the diagnosis (using a special salivary sample kit) may be requested by the Health Protection Agency after the disease has been notified

Action
- paracetamol or ibuprofen may ease the discomfort
- maintain fluid intake
- acidic fruit juices may intensify the pain and should be avoided
- advise – infectious for five days after the onset of swelling
- complete 'notification of infectious diseases' form
- patients may ask whether vulnerable contacts who have not previously received two doses of mumps vaccine should be vaccinated. Unfortunately it will not provide protection against this infection, although it may be a good time to persuade them to be vaccinated

Refer to doctor
- if symptoms of meningitis, abdominal or testicular pain are present
- if patient is pregnant

Earache

History	• duration of pain
	• fever
	• deafness
	• discharge
	• recent swimming
	• previous attacks (how treated and what happened)
	• immunocompromised
Examination	• canal for inflammation, foreign body, discharge or swelling (general or local, e.g. boil)
	• eardrum to assess colour, dullness, perforation, bulging/ retracted, fluid level
Tests	• if there is copious discharge, take ear swab (being careful not to puncture the drum)
Action	• depends on diagnosis – *see* subsections:
	– otitis media
	– otitis externa
	– boil in ear canal
	– eustachian catarrh

Otitis media

Otitis media causes pain, deafness and sometimes fever, vomiting and loss of balance. The eardrum is red. It may be bulging or a discharge may be present. If the history is suggestive but the drum cannot be seen (e.g. because of wax) it is safest to assume that otitis media is present. Pink eardrums are to be expected if other membranes are inflamed (e.g. conjunctivitis, red throat), or after crying. Antibiotics are not necessary for these patients.

Action	• recommend adequate analgesia with ibuprofen and/or paracetamol

- give antibiotics if immunocompromised, or severe malaise with fever and vomiting

- otherwise, explain that antibiotics are not helpful for the majority of patients with otitis media; 60% of patients will be pain-free within 24 h, whether or not they take antibiotics, and the chances of experiencing a side-effect from the antibiotic are greater than the chances of benefiting. Reassure that ear infections very rarely cause permanent hearing damage

- if patient/parent is unhappy with this advice, consider offering a delayed antibiotic prescription for use if there is no improvement within 48 h

Prescription/OTC
- ibuprofen and/or paracetamol

- if antibiotic indicated: amoxicillin for 3 to 5 days, clarithromycin if the patient is allergic to penicillin

Caution
- patients with otitis media should be made aware that flying or diving may cause severe pain and perforation

- severe infections may cause temporary deafness by perforation of the eardrum, which will usually heal in a few weeks

Refer to doctor
- make appointment if:

  - hearing does not return to normal within 14 days

  - more than six episodes of otitis media per year

References

- Bertin L, Pons G, d'Athis P *et al.* (1996) A randomized double blind multicentre controlled trial of ibuprofen versus acetaminophen and placebo for symptoms of acute otitis media in children. *Fundam Clin Pharmacol* **10**: 387–92.
- Cates C (1999) An evidence based approach to reducing antibiotic use in children with acute otitis media: controlled before and after study. *BMJ* **318**: 715–16.
- Glasziou P, Hayem M and Del Mar C (2003) Antibiotic versus placebo for acute otitis media in children (Cochrane review). *The Cochrane Library, Issue 4, 2003.* Update Software, Oxford.

Otitis externa

This is a form of infected eczema which causes itchy discomfort rather than pain. It may follow inappropriate probing of the ear with a hairgrip or cotton bud, or the presence of a foreign body. It may be recurrent. Insertion of the auriscope is often uncomfortable. The canal looks irregular, red or moist, perhaps with discharge.

Test • take swab if there is copious discharge

Action • recommend cotton wool and Vaseline to keep shampoo and shower gel out of inflamed ears while showering or washing hair

• recommend avoiding swimming while ear is inflamed

Prescription/OTC • if there is purulent discharge after swimming, give Otosporin eardrops for 7 days

• otherwise consider Earcalm (OTC) or Otomize

Refer to doctor • if persistent/recurrent symptoms, for consideration of ENT referral

Reference
• Bojrab DI, Bruderly T and Abdulrazzak Y (1996) Otitis externa. *Otolaryngol Clin North Am* **5**: 761–82.

Boil in ear canal

This causes a localised red swelling in the canal, often with unilateral deafness and severe pain on insertion of the auriscope.

Action • give oral flucloxacillin for 5 days, or erythromycin/ clarithromycin if the patient is allergic to penicillin

• warn the patient that the ear may discharge

Eustachian catarrh

The hearing is impaired and the ear is intermittently uncomfortable. The eardrum may appear normal, retracted or bulging. A fluid level may be seen behind the drum, which is not inflamed.

Action	• explain that the eardrum is a sensitive structure that hurts when the pressure changes. When catarrh blocks the eustachian tube, changes in atmospheric pressure cause earache that comes and goes
	• ask patient to try to 'pop' the ears
Prescription/OTC	• paracetamol for children
	• menthol and eucalyptus inhalations for adults
	• pseudoephedrine may give temporary relief, but *see* the contraindications and cautions in the Formulary
Refer to doctor	• if not improving after two weeks

Colds and 'flu

Be aware that although most patients with a 'flu-like illness will indeed have a simple viral infection, there are many rare diseases that give the same initial symptoms. If the history has some odd features, or if the symptoms have been going on rather too long for a simple cold, then ask open general questions to see if there could be an alternative source of infection (such as the urinary tract).

History	• duration
	• fever
	• foreign travel
	• joint and muscle pains
	• sinus pain
	• earache
	• productive cough

- urinary symptoms
- lactating
- what medicine has been tried
- immunocompromised
- travel to tropical region in last 12 months

Examination
- ears
- throat
- chest

Tests
- none

Action
- if mastitis/sinusitis/otitis media/cough with crackles in chest, refer to relevant section
- if not, explain the nature of viral infections and stress that antibiotics will not help

Prescription/OTC
- paracetamol or ibuprofen for sore throat and headache
- steam or menthol inhalations for nasal congestion
- saline nose drops for babies
- chlorphenamine at night may help congestion
- pseudoephedrine (*see* cautions in Formulary) is a non-drowsy decongestant
- there is some (controversial) evidence that echinacea preparations, zinc lozenges and high-dose vitamin C may shorten the duration of colds. Suggest that the patient discusses this with a pharmacist

Refer to doctor
- if the symptoms do not fit comfortably with a diagnosis of a cold or 'flu
- if feverish, and the patient has recently travelled to tropical region

Caution	• do not confuse with hayfever (no fever, recurrent spring symptoms)
	• if high fever, *see also* cautions in fever section, page 30

References

• Melchart D, Linde K, Fischer P *et al.* (2004) Echinacea for preventing and treating the common cold (Cochrane review). *The Cochrane Library, Issue 4, 2004.* Update Software, Oxford.
• Mossad S, Macknin M and Medendorp S (1996) Zinc gluconate lozenges for treating the common cold. A randomized, double-blind, placebo-controlled study. *Ann Intern Med* **125**: 81–8.
• Douglas RM, Hemila H, D'Souza R, Chalker EB and B Treacy B (2004) Vitamin C for preventing and treating the common cold (Cochrane review). *The Cochrane Library, Issue 4, 2004.* Update Software, Oxford.

Sinusitis

This condition is very difficult to diagnose because the traditional symptoms and signs are unreliable.

History	• duration: relapsing symptoms after initial improvement suggest secondary bacterial infection
	• fever
	• facial pain: worse on bending forwards
	• purulent nasal discharge
	• previous episodes: how were they treated?
	• immunocompromised
Examination	• there are no reliable signs of sinusitis, but check for other sites of infection:
	– throat (post-nasal discharge)
	– ears
	– localised swelling on face
Tests	• none

Action • avoid smoky atmospheres

Prescription/OTC • analgesia with paracetamol or ibuprofen

• steam inhalations with menthol and eucalyptus

• antibiotics are of marginal benefit. In severe or persistent cases, or immunocompromised patients, consider amoxicillin for 7 days (or doxycycline if the patient is allergic to penicillin)

Refer to doctor • same day if:

– severe illness

– localised swelling around the eyes, cheeks or on forehead (may indicate intracranial infection or abscess)

Refer to dentist • if unilateral maxillary sinusitis (may be secondary to dental infection)

Reference

• Williams JW, Aguilar C, Cornell J *et al.* (2004) Antibiotics for acute maxillary sinusitis (Cochrane Review). *The Cochrane Library, Issue 4, 2004.* Update Software, Oxford.

Cough

History • duration

• dry/productive/wheezy

• daytime/night-time/on exertion

• loss of voice

• colour of sputum – bloodstained (haemoptysis)

• fever

• chest pain

• breathlessness

• previous similar episodes (how treated and what happened)

- known chest problems
- smoking (amount, duration)
- immunocompromised

Examination
- cyanosis
- breathlessness
- confusion
- fever
- respiratory rate
- crackles in chest (and where located)
- wheezing
- subcostal/intercostal recession especially in babies
- ears and throat in children (otitis media and tonsillitis may coexist)

Tests
- peak expiratory flow if wheezing heard in adult or child over 5 years (*see* section on acute asthma, page 24)
- sputum culture is unhelpful, except in special cases (e.g. cystic fibrosis or bronchiectasis) or if tuberculosis is suspected

Action
- adequate fluid intake
- steam or menthol and eucalyptus inhalations two to three times a day
- stop smoking (includes parents of coughing child)
- antibiotics are not indicated for most patients with coughs, but should be given if:
  - sputum brown or bloodstained (NB possibility of cancer, may need X-ray/referral)
  - severe malaise
  - crackles in the chest
  - history of chronic obstructive pulmonary disease (COPD)/bronchiectasis

– smoker aged over 55 years

– immunocompromised

Prescription/OTC • if antibiotics indicated, give amoxicillin for 7 days (or erythromycin/clarithromycin if allergic to penicillin)

• if not responding to amoxicillin and further antibiotics indicated, add doxycycline or change to erythromycin/ clarithromycin

• simple linctus or pholcodine may be helpful (though not curative) to soothe an irritating cough

• pseudoephedrine may be helpful if there is marked nasal congestion (but *see* cautions in Formulary)

• if wheezing in child under 5 years, salbutamol via Aerochamber (can be used with paediatric mask for children of 2 years or younger): 100 µg single dose four times a day

• if wheezing in older child or adult:

– bronchodilator: inhaled salbutamol 200 µg four times a day for up to 1 week

– if not better or still needing bronchodilator after 1 week, recommend review appointment with doctor

Refer to doctor • urgently if:

– baby with rapid respirations, intercostal/subcostal recession, wheezes or crackles (may be bronchiolitis)

– cyanosis

– mental confusion

– very unwell or distressed

– peak expiratory flow below 75% of predicted value

– one-sided chest pain, worse on coughing or deep breathing (suggests pleurisy, pneumonia, pulmonary embolism or pneumothorax)

• make appointment if persistent or recurrent symptoms

Caution
- danger signs are moderate to severe breathlessness, distress, chest pain, cyanosis, pallor, subcostal/intercostal recession and raised respiratory rate in children

- beware of asthmatics who look ill, and have passed from the wheezy to the non-wheezy phase. Experienced asthmatics will tell you how bad they are, and usually know what is needed from previous episodes

References

- Geelhoed GC, Turner J and Macdonald WB (1996) Efficacy of a small single dose of oral dexamethasone for outpatient croup: a double blind placebo controlled clinical trial. *BMJ* **313**: 140–2.
- Lentino JR and Lucks DA (1987) Nonvalue of sputum culture in the management of lower respiratory tract infections. *J Clin Microbiol* **25**: 758–62.
- Mills GD, Oehley MR and Arrol B (2005) Effectiveness of beta lactam antibiotics compared with antibiotics active against atypical pathogens in non-severe community-acquired pneumonia: meta-analysis. *BMJ* **330**: 456–60.
- Smucny J, Fahey T, Becker L and Glazier R (2004) Antibiotics for acute bronchitis (Cochrane Review). *The Cochrane Library, Issue 4, 2004*. Update Software, Oxford.

Box 1.1   Notes on cough

Cough is a very common presenting symptom, other symptoms may accompany it and help to make a diagnosis. The patient may present because the cough is persistent or interferes with sleep, or because of anxiety that infection is 'going to the chest'. Quite often a friend or relative has suggested that the patient should seek medical help. Mothers may fear that their children will choke in the night.

Cough may be due to:

- infection. This is the *commonest* cause of a cough in primary care. Most are viral but some are caused by primary or secondary infection with bacteria. Loss of voice suggests laryngitis, for which antibiotics are ineffective
- physical and chemical stimuli, e.g. cold air, cigarette smoke
- circulatory problems. A persistent dry cough in the elderly, with crackles at the lung bases, is likely to be due to heart failure. Dry cough and sometimes haemoptysis following sudden chest pain may be due to pulmonary embolism
- cancer. A persistent cough in a smoker, associated with chest pain, haemoptysis or weight loss, is suspicious
- iatrogenic causes. Cough is commonly caused by angiotensin-converting enzyme inhibitors (drug names ending in '-april')
- habit

continued opposite

A persistent or relapsing cough may occur in:

- asthmatics (young children may present with cough without wheezing)
- heavy smokers (but beware cancer)
- small children with catarrh
- whooping cough (rare, thanks to immunisation)
- *Mycoplasma pneumoniae*, an unusual type of infection which occurs in cycles of 3–5 years. It causes a cough which may last for three months. It is sensitive to erythromycin/clarithromycin or doxycycline, but not amoxicillin. A two-week course is necessary
- tuberculosis

After a viral infection the cough may last for some weeks. Patients may expect proprietary cough medicines to cure the cough and come for something stronger because brand X 'hasn't worked'. They need gentle re-education. Simple linctus or pholcodine may be helpful (although not curative) to soothe an irritating cough.

References
- Cornford CS, Morgan M and Ridsdale L (1993) Why do mothers consult when their children cough? *Fam Pract* **10**: 193–6.
- Johnson G and Helman C (2004) Remedy or cure? Lay beliefs about over-the-counter medicines for coughs and colds. *Br J Gen Pract* **54**: 98–102.
- Zola IK (1973) Pathways to the doctor: from person to patient. *Soc Sci Med* **7**: 677–89.

Croup

A viral infection of children aged between 3 months and 5 years.

History
- cough (often 'brassy' or 'barking')
- crowing noise on inspiration (stridor, worse at night)

Examination
- breathless
- respiratory rate
- listen to chest (usually normal)
- examine throat

Action
- explain nature of illness
- steam inhalations are often used but their effectiveness is not proven

Refer to doctor
- immediately for consideration of single dose of oral steroid

Reference

- Russell K, Wiebe N, Saenz A *et al*. (2003) Glucocorticoids for croup (Cochrane Review). *The Cochrane Library, Issue 2, 2003*. Update Software, Oxford.

Acute asthma

Nurses vary in their confidence in dealing with asthma. Asthma specialist nurses will be able to manage more severe cases.

History
- known asthmatic
- previous admissions to hospital
- duration of symptoms:
  - wheeze
  - breathlessness
  - cough, especially at night
  - tightness in the chest
- present and previous medication
- smoker (if a child, do parents or carers smoke?)
- fever
- chest pain

Examination
- ability to complete sentences
- pallor/cyanosis
- respiratory rate
- pulse rate
- subcostal/intercostal recession

- listen to chest for wheezes/crackles (crackles suggest bacterial infection; *see* cough, page 19)

Tests
- peak expiratory flow (PEF) (Caution: *see* Box 1.2)

- compare with predicted rate from charts (*see* Figure 1.1 and Table 1.1), and the patient's usual rate

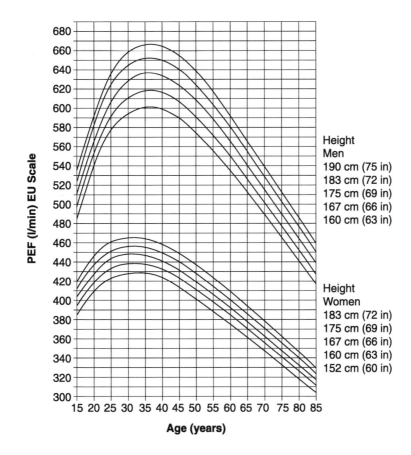

Figure 1.1 Peak expiratory flow – normal values in adults. Peak flow chart reproduced with permission of Clement Clarke International and adapted for use with EN13826/EU scale peak flow meters. From Nunn AJ and Gregg I (1989) New regression equations for predicting peak expiratory flow in adults. *BMJ* **298**: 1068–70.

Table 1.1 Peak expiratory flow – normal values in children. Normal PEF values in children correlate best with height; with increasing age, larger differences occur between the sexes. These predicted values are based on the formulae given in Cotes JE and Leathart GL (1993) *Lung Function* (4e) Blackwell, Oxford, adapted for EU scale-Mini-Wright peak flow meters by Clement Clarke

Height (m)	Height (ft)	Predicted EU PEF (l/min)	Height (m)	Height (ft)	Predicted EU PEF (l/min)
0.85	2´ 9´´	87	1.30	4´ 3´´	212
0.90	2´ 11´´	95	1.35	4´ 5´´	233
0.95	3´ 1´´	104	1.40	4´ 7´´	254
1.00	3´ 3´´	115	1.45	4´ 9´´	276
1.05	3´ 5´´	127	1.50	4´ 11´´	299
1.10	3´ 7´´	141	1.55	5´ 1´´	323
1.15	3´ 9´´	157	1.60	5´ 3´´	346
1.20	3´ 11´´	174	1.65	5´ 5´´	370
1.25	4´ 1´´	192	1.70	5´ 7´´	393

Action

Follow the British Thoracic Society (BTS) guidelines, which can be found in Chapter 3 of the *BNF*:

Adults and children over 5 years with PEF greater than 75% of expected value:

- give usual inhaled bronchodilator. Check PEF afterwards
- check inhaler technique
- consider commencing inhaled beclometasone, or ensure that the patient is taking an adequate dose of inhaled corticosteroid
- asthma specialists may consider adding a long-acting beta-agonist (LABA)
- consider prescribing peak flow meter if patient does not already have one
- recommend recording the results on a chart
- advise the patient to seek further help from the most appropriate NHS agency if the asthma worsens despite the increase in treatment
- follow up in asthma clinic after 1–2 weeks for review of long-term treatment

Children 5 years and younger with mild symptoms

- try usual bronchodilator or, if uncooperative, nebulised salbutamol 2.5 mg

- observe, assess effect, listen to the chest again

- consider commencing inhaled beclometasone, or ensure that the patient is taking an adequate dose of inhaled corticosteroid

- continue inhaled bronchodilator, but ensure adequate technique

- if inadequate, consider changing the inhaler delivery system, e.g. using an Aerochamber or changing to a breath-actuated device

- advise parents to seek further medical help if the asthma worsens: child more distressed, breathing faster, wheezing more, recession

- review in asthma clinic after 1–7 days depending on severity and parental confidence in dealing with asthma

Refer to doctor
- immediately if:
  - silent chest
  - cyanosis
  - exhaustion
  - slow pulse
  - PEF below 75% of predicted rate
  - child: distressed; respiratory rate over 40/minute; recession; widespread wheezes
  - chest pain (suggests asthma is complicated by pleurisy, pneumothorax or pulmonary embolus)

Caution
Peak flow meters have recently been changed to comply with EU regulations, and unfortunately the scales on the two types of meter do not correspond. *See* Box 1.2.

> **Box 1.2   Changes to peak flow meters**
>
> In 2004 a new EU standard was introduced for peak flow meters. The new EN 13826 meters are recognisable by the bright yellow band which carries the measurements. Unfortunately, the scale of the new meters gives readings that may be very different from the old type, up to 50 l/min lower in the middle of the range.
>
> This may cause confusion between patients who may have the old meters at home and professionals who have the EU type in their consulting rooms. Conversion charts and normal ranges are available at www.peakflow.com.
>
> There is a particular problem with assessing adolescents, because the expected peak flow values are very different for the same patient on the children's and adults' charts.

Fever

History
- duration
- degree (if accurate thermometer used)
- any other symptoms
- headache
- sore throat/cold
- cough
- dysuria/frequency
- vomiting/diarrhoea
- abdominal/loin pain
- rash
- drowsiness/photophobia
- lactating
- travel to tropical area in last 12 months
- immunocompromised

Examination	• ears
(as suggested	• throat
by symptoms)	• cervical lymph nodes
	• chest
	• rash (beware the petechial rash of meningitis)
	• neck stiffness (e.g. can a child kiss his knees)
	• breasts in lactating women
	• any painful area (e.g. sinuses, abdomen)

Tests

• test urine for nitrites, protein and blood if cause of fever not obvious (to avoid contaminating the whole sample, pour a little urine on the test strip)

• send mid-stream urine (MSU) for culture if test positive or any urinary symptoms

Action

• ample fluid intake

• avoid over-strenuous activity

• paracetamol/ibuprofen as needed to relieve discomfort

• assume a viral cause if no other clues, fever less than 7 days' duration and generally well

• otherwise give treatment appropriate to cause

• reduce anxiety about fever, by explaining that it is produced by the body's immune system in response to an infection, is unlikely to cause any harm and may aid recovery

Refer to doctor

• immediately if:

   – photophobia, neck stiffness, drowsiness or petechial rash

   – appears very unwell

   – unexplained fever lasting more than 7 days

   – immunocompromised

   – travel to tropical area in last 12 months

Caution
- mastitis may cause 'flu-like symptoms in a breastfeeding woman with only minimal signs in the breast

- malaria may cause an illness indistinguishable from 'flu and taking malaria prophylaxis may not prevent malaria. If patient has visited an area where falciparum malaria occurs, a 'test and treat' strategy is recommended, where empirical treatment is given without waiting for the test result

- meningitis in its early stages is impossible to distinguish from a simple viral infection. Diarrhoea and vomiting may cause confusion with gastroenteritis, and the rash of meningococcal septicaemia may initially appear macular and blanch on pressure. Ensure that the patient/parent knows that they should contact the appropriate NHS service if symptoms worsen

- fever with no associated other symptoms or signs of a focus of infection may require thorough investigation in hospital to discover the hidden cause

Hay fever

History
- April to August
- frequent sneezing
- blocked nose
- red, itchy, watery eyes
- dry, sore throat
- wheeze, chest tightness, cough
- has patient tried any OTC treatment?
- with what effect?

Examination
- none

Tests
- none

Action
- advise patient to avoid long grass, fragrant flowers and newly mown lawns
- there is no evidence to support the standard advice to sleep with windows closed

Prescription/OTC
- one or a combination of:
  - antihistamines: non-sedative, e.g. loratadine, cetirizine or fexofenadine, or sedative, e.g. chlorphenamine
  - eyedrops: sodium cromoglicate
  - nose spray: beclometasone aqueous nasal spray

Refer to doctor
- if symptoms persist after various combinations of the above have been tried

Nosebleeds (epistaxis)

History
- duration
- extent of blood loss
- trauma, including nose-picking
- symptoms of sinusitis
- cold
- hayfever
- foreign body
- offensive discharge (may indicate a foreign body)
- previous episodes
- history of anaemia, leukaemia, coagulation problems
- anticoagulant/antiplatelet therapy (including aspirin)

Examination
- which nostril?
- evidence of infection inside nostril
- check for foreign body, if appropriate

- adults may expect you to check their blood pressure, but the chance of finding hypertension is not increased. Be aware, though, that the stress of the nosebleed may temporarily elevate blood pressure

Tests
- consider FBC if severe/recurrent

Action
- advise pinching middle third of nose, just below end of nasal bone, continuously for 10 minutes

- if infection seen, prescribe sodium fusidate ointment for 7 days

- if sinusitis present, refer to relevant section

Refer to doctor
- urgently if:
  - bleeding does not stop within 20 minutes
  - blood disorder known or suspected
  - patient taking anticoagulant/antiplatelet medication
- routinely: if recurrent problems

References

- Herkner H, Laggner A, Mullner M *et al.* (2000) Hypertension in patients presenting with epistaxis. *Ann Emerg Med* **35**: 126–30.
- Ruddy J, Proops D, Pearman K *et al.* (1991) Management of epistaxis in children. *Int J Pediatr Otorhinolaryngol* **21**: 139–42.

2 Head, neck and back

Headache

History

- duration
- onset: sudden/gradual
- time of day
- linked to menstrual cycle/combined oral contraceptive
- quality: sharp/like a pressure or band/throbbing
- site
- associated symptoms:
  - visual disturbance
  - gut symptoms, e.g. nausea/diarrhoea/dyspepsia/heartburn
  - fever
  - cough
  - sinus problems
  - neck pain
  - neurological symptoms, e.g. sensory disturbance, double vision, inco-ordination
- any known triggers
- anything that worsens pain, e.g. bending over, coughing
- previous recurrent headaches
- recent head injury
- recent stress/worries/depression/disturbed sleep
- treatment tried and effect
- we all get headaches – what is different about this one?

Examination

- observe the face for signs of swelling or infection
- neck movements/tenderness

- blood pressure (has to be really high – above 200/115 mmHg – to cause headache)

Tests
- take blood for erythrocyte sedimentation rate (ESR) in patients aged over 50 years with onset of headaches within the last three months

Action
- if cause is obvious, reassure and explain
- suggest simple analgesics, e.g. ibuprofen (most people have only tried paracetamol)

Refer to doctor
- immediately if suspicious features:
  - sudden 'thunderclap' headache
  - any other neurological symptoms
  - suspicion of meningitis
  - regular user of analgesics, particularly those containing codeine, which may cause 'analgesic headaches'
  - patient over 50 years with unexplained headaches
  - focal migraine (including migraine with aura, which is now a contraindication to the combined oral contraceptive (COC)) in patient taking COC

Refer to optometrist
If patient concerned about cerebral tumour – explain that they can check for papilloedema, a sign of raised intracranial pressure

Caution (all rare)
- temporal arteritis (*see* Box 2.1)
- meningitis
- acute glaucoma
- carbon monoxide poisoning
- subarachnoid haemorrhage (sudden severe pain)
- cerebral tumour (headache on waking, often worse on bending/coughing, often with associated neurological disturbance which may be mild)

Box 2.1   Temporal arteritis

This causes inflammation in small- to medium-sized arteries. It is more common over the age of 50 years, but may affect younger people. The headache is severe, often associated with tenderness of the scalp and sometimes aching of the jaw muscles on eating. There may be associated weakness of other muscles with morning stiffness, aches and weight loss. It is significant because it may cause sudden occlusion of important blood vessels, resulting in blindness, stroke or myocardial infarction, so patients in whom it is suspected should be referred urgently to a doctor. A raised ESR will help in confirming the diagnosis. Long-term oral steroid treatment is needed.

Box 2.2   Migraine

Early symptoms such as excessive tiredness, yawning, pallor, visual disturbances and restlessness may start many hours before the headache. The headache is often severe, throbbing or bursting, unilateral, associated with nausea or other gut symptoms, and may last more than 24 h.

Migraine is caused by abnormal changes in the size of the blood vessels in the head and neck, although the initial event that starts an attack probably occurs in the brain, in the hypothalamus. A wide variety of factors are known to trigger migraine:

- stress
- light
- menstrual cycle hormones
- diet (e.g. citrus fruit, cheese, alcohol). Dietary factors are often suspected but rarely found, and searching too hard may divert attention away from more likely factors such as stress
- starvation
- noise
- sleep disturbance
- hypoxia

For most people the attacks seem to be multifactorial, and it is often not possible to identify any one trigger, which either always causes migraine or, when avoided, stops all attacks. Whatever the cause, the final part of the sequence of events leading to symptoms involves the neurotransmitter 5-hydroxytryptamine (serotonin, 5-HT). Many new

continued overleaf

anti-migraine drugs are 5-HT agonists, which are used to treat attacks, not prevent them. Although these drugs are effective, they should only be prescribed when simpler and safer methods of treatment have failed.

Patients often know a remedy that works for them, for example a cup of tea, a lie-down in a quiet room and a short sleep. When this is either impractical or ineffective, then drugs have a role. Simple analgesics work for many sufferers, but they must be taken early in the attack. If there is associated nausea it is important to treat this as well, with an anti-emetic such as domperidone.

Migraine associated with difficulty in reading, particularly in children or young people, may respond to colour tinting of spectacles. Referral to an optometrist for an intuitive colorimeter test may both help the migraine and (importantly) improve educational potential.

Adults with frequent dyspepsia or heartburn should be referred to a doctor for investigation. If the presence of *Helicobacter pylori* is confirmed, eradication therapy may abolish the migraine as well as the gut symptoms.

If these measures do not control the migraine, refer to the GP for consideration of specific anti-migraine therapy. If attacks are frequent (e.g. once a week) preventative treatment may be considered, although there is no ideal drug for this.

References
- Bal SK and Hollingworth GR (2005) 10-minute consultation: headache. *BMJ* **330**: 346.
- British Association for the Study of Headache (BASH). www.bash.org.uk/bash/guidelines.htm
- Gasbarrini A, De LA, Fiore G *et al.* (1998) Beneficial effects of *Helicobacter pylori* eradication on migraine. *Hepatogastroenterology* **45**: 765–70.
- Machlachlan A, Yale S and Wilkins A (1993) Open trial of subjective precision tinting: a follow-up of 55 patients. *Ophthalmic Physiol Optic* **13**: 175–8.

Notes on headache

Only about 10% of headaches have a treatable cause. Less than 0.5% are serious. Severe headaches are not necessarily the ones of greater concern. The commonest cause of headache is stress. Features of a suspicious headache are shown in Table 2.1.

Table 2.1 Features of a suspicious headache

Reassuring	Suspicious
On the top of my head	Always there when I wake up
Like a band around my head	Hurts more when I cough or bend over
It can last all day	Localised
It can come on at any time	Sudden onset
I've had it for years on and off	Associated with other symptoms:
	• visual, especially in elderly
	• nausea
	• weakness
	• numbness, pins and needles
	• inco-ordination

Dizziness

History
- duration
- nature: spinning (vertigo) or faint feeling
- associated symptoms:
    - nausea
    - earache
    - deafness
    - tinnitus
    - viral infection
- previous episodes
- recent head injury
- medication (e.g. antihypertensives)

Examination
- ears
- blood pressure (usually taken with the patient sitting, but also standing if the symptoms mainly occur on standing)
- pallor

Tests	• FBC if anaemia suspected
	• otherwise none

Advice	• dizziness is common and often accompanies viral infections
	• will usually settle, but may sometimes take several weeks
	• sit and stand slowly; rest
	• driving or other critical tasks may be affected

Prescription	• if true vertigo, prochlorperazine (buccal form available OTC)

Refer to doctor
- urgently if:
  - neurological symptoms or signs
  - headache
  - deafness, especially if new and unilateral
  - previous ear surgery
  - recent head injury
- routinely if:
  - on antihypertensive treatment and blood pressure is low
  - persistent/recurrent symptoms
  - elderly

Neck pain

History
- duration
- injury, e.g. whiplash
- sore throat
- is patient worried about meningitis?
- occupation (e.g. checkout/keyboard operator)

	• onset: sudden/known trigger/gradual
	• psychosocial stress
Examination	• cervical lymph nodes
	• neck movements and their limits
	• posture

| *Tests* | • none |

Action	• analgesia, e.g. ibuprofen or paracetamol
	• local heat
	• gentle exercises – give leaflet
	• attention to posture
	• consider manipulation or acupuncture
	• reassure about meningitis

| *Refer to doctor* | • if severe pain, or not responding to simple analgesics in 4–5 days |

| *Caution* | • instantaneous onset of neck pain and stiffness may be due to subarachnoid haemorrhage |

Back pain

History	• occupation
	• onset: gradual/sudden
	• while lifting
	• duration/previous episodes
	• radiation to leg – especially below the knee
	• numbness/tingling of leg or peri-anal area
	• difficulty passing urine
	• abdominal pain

- coldness/cyanosis of legs
- weight loss/malaise
- steroid therapy
- psychosocial stress

Examination
- ask patient to show site of pain
- observe the back for signs of muscle spasm
- spinal movement (flexion/extension/rotation)
- spinal tenderness
- if leg symptoms, check straight leg raising – record angles

Tests
- not necessary. Patients who expect an X-ray should be gently told that it will be of no help in finding the cause of their pain, and that the dose of radiation required is 120 times that of a chest X-ray

Action
- reassure the patient that most back pain is not serious and will get better without treatment. The patient's emotional health plays a major part in the resolution of their back pain, and it is very important that health professionals convey a positive attitude from the beginning
- encourage gentle mobilisation (activity within the limits of pain as soon as possible)
- analgesics relieve pain and muscle spasm. If the patient pays prescription charges, ibuprofen and paracetamol are cheaper if bought OTC. Combination analgesics containing codeine are also available OTC, but to obtain additional analgesia from codeine it is necessary to take at least 25 mg per dose, and many common combinations contain suboptimal doses. Suggest that the patient discusses this with the pharmacist:
  - ibuprofen
  - paracetamol
  - dihydrocodeine, if necessary (NB this may cause constipation, which may be difficult to manage when patient has back pain)

- give back-care leaflet
- recommend manipulation if available/affordable

Refer to doctor
- urgently if:
    - numbness/tingling in peri-anal area or difficulty passing urine (extremely rare)
    - sudden onset of severe pain with abdominal pain, discoloration of legs or stiffness (possible dissection of aortic aneurysm)
    - analgesics ineffective (diazepam may be helpful if muscle spasm is prominent)
- routinely if:
    - severe symptoms or sciatica (pain/numbness/tingling in one leg extending below the knee)
    - aged <20years, >55 years, or taking oral corticosteroids

Caution
- unilateral pain over renal area may have a renal cause: arrange urine dipstick test and MSU for culture
- instantaneous onset of back pain and stiffness without an obvious trigger may be due to subarachnoid haemorrhage
- back pain may be caused by abdominal pathology such as an aortic aneurysm
- night pain, weight loss, malaise and/or spinal tenderness suggest spinal metastases

References

- Kendrick D, Fielding K, Bentley E *et al.* (2001) Radiography of the lumbar spine in primary care patients with low back pain: randomized controlled trial. *BMJ* **322**: 400–5.
- No authors listed (1998) Managing acute low back pain. *Drug Ther Bull* **36**: 93–5.
- Vickers A (2000) Recent advances: complementary medicine. *BMJ* **321**: 683–6.

3 Eyes

Sore eyes

History
- duration
- contacts (e.g. sibling)
- associated cold symptoms
- any problem with vision
- discharge
- diabetes
- previous eye problems, e.g. iritis
- history of trauma/foreign body/drilling or grinding, especially metal
- contact lens use

Examination
In uncomplicated conjunctivitis no examination may be necessary.
- normal visual acuity is the most helpful sign in excluding a serious eye condition
- discharge
- redness
- bilateral or unilateral
- pupils equal and react to light
- look for foreign body (evert eyelid), especially if symptoms unilateral
- scales at roots of eyelashes (blepharitis)
- lids (stye, meibomian cyst, cellulitis)
- painful clusters of spots around eye (possible shingles)

Tests

- take bacterial and chlamydial swabs if persistent or recurrent symptoms. Remember that it is necessary to press firmly with a chlamydial swab

- stain with fluorescein if unilateral/history of trauma/ recent use of power tools (but do not use with contact lens *in situ*)

Action –
depends
on cause

1 Infective conjunctivitis: sore eyes, red conjunctival membranes, usually with discharge. May be unilateral, especially in early stages. Check for scales on roots of eyelashes, if present *see* blepharitis.

Viral conjunctivitis is very likely if symptoms are mild and concurrent with an upper respiratory tract infection, in which case no treatment is needed other than wiping the eyes with cotton wool soaked in cooled boiled water. Otherwise:

- administer chloramphenicol eyedrops as often as possible (every 3 h ideally initially). Ointment may be easier to apply in babies. Drops are now available OTC for adults and children aged two and over

- if severe, apply ointment at night also (treat only the infected eye(s))

- if contact lenses are worn, suggest that they are cleaned and not used until the eye has healed, advise patient to see optometrist if symptoms are recurrent

- advise about infectiousness, use own face cloth and towel

- although the Health Protection Agency (HPA) does not recommend exclusion, schools and nurseries prefer that children with conjunctivitis do not attend until discharge has gone

2 Allergic conjunctivitis: longer history, itchy inflammation, frequent 'attacks', hay fever symptoms, watering rather than discharge

- avoid triggers, e.g. mascara

- use sodium cromoglicate eyedrops four times a day (OTC)

3 Dry eyes: older patients more commonly affected, eyes feel gritty but look normal, vision unaffected

- artificial tears help if used often (hypromellose, available OTC)

4 Blepharitis: conjunctivitis with scales at roots of eyelashes

- apply chloramphenicol eye ointment
- remove scales by applying warm compresses, then wiping lids twice daily for two weeks with cotton wool dipped in diluted baby shampoo, or a pinch of sodium bicarbonate in a cup of cooled, boiled water. Long-term lid hygiene should be recommended

Refer to doctor • same day if:

  - abnormal shape or reaction of pupils to light

  - reduced visual acuity

  - foreign body in eye or under eyelid which you cannot remove with irrigation/moist cotton bud

  - persistent/recurrent symptoms

  - severe inflammation

  - shingles/herpes simplex suspected

  - any abnormality seen using fluorescein

Caution • iritis (reduced visual acuity, unequal/irregular pupils, photophobia)

- *Chlamydia* (pale bumps on inner lids – neonates are most commonly affected)

- herpes (cold sores, shingles)

- contact lens problems (consult optometrist)

Reference
- Rietveld R, van Weert CPM, ter Riet G *et al.* (2003) Diagnostic impact of signs and symptoms in acute infectious conjunctivitis: systematic literature search. *BMJ* **327**: 789.

Subconjunctival haemorrhage

This may sometimes be confused with conjunctivitis. It causes a sudden uniform red area in the eye with a sharp edge. You should be able to see the posterior margin. There is no discomfort, discharge or deterioration in vision. Patients often worry that the haemorrhage may be a sign of high blood pressure. Although there is no evidence for this, checking the blood pressure (BP) will reassure the patient.

Styes

History	• how long present?
	• has it discharged?
Examination	• any associated conjunctivitis or cellulitis?
Tests	• none
Action	• none may be necessary if resolving or discharged
	• otherwise give chloramphenicol eye ointment
	• warn that styes are infectious; care with hygiene
	• if there is any sign of cellulitis of the eyelid, give antibiotics (*see* page 66)

4 Skin and mouth

Nurses often find skin problems daunting at first. Remember two important principles, which apply equally to all types of minor illness:

- find out and address the patient's agenda
- take a good history

Caution
- in darkly pigmented skin, it is difficult to assess the degree of inflammation

It may be helpful to compare the patient's rash with pictures; Dermnet (www.dermnetnz.org) is a good online resource, or use one of the many books available.

Reference

- Ankrett V and Williams I (1999) *Quick Reference Atlas of Dermatology*. MSL, Tunbridge Wells.

Rashes

History
- unwell: fever/malaise
- duration
- did all spots appear at same time, or sequentially?
- is rash constant, spreading, or coming and going?
- distribution
- any contacts who are itching?
- possibility of pregnancy?
- on any medication?

Examination
- site and distribution (remember to look in the mouth)

- are the spots:
  - clearly defined and separate (discrete)?
  - wheal-like (irregular, raised, blotchy)?
  - flat (macules) or raised (papules)?
- are burrows visible on the hands?
- are blisters present?

Tests
- none

Action/referral
- *see* different diagnoses

Acute itchy rashes

Acute itchy rashes may be caused by:

- chickenpox
- urticaria
- scabies
- eczema (*see* page 55)
- fungal infections (*see* page 58)

Chickenpox

- separate itchy papules at different stages of development, turning into blisters
- fever and malaise, more marked in adults

Action
- calamine or crotamiton lotion OTC (keep in fridge) are often used to reduce itching
- perhaps antihistamines – chlorphenamine is useful for children at night because of its sedative action
- inform contacts who are pregnant or immunocompromised

Refer to doctor   • urgently if:

- immunocompromised

- breathless/confused/severe headache

- pregnant

- less than 4 weeks after childbirth

- a baby aged under 4 weeks

Caution   • may rarely be complicated by pneumonia or encephalitis; pregnant women are at highest risk

• secondary bacterial infection is often suspected when chickenpox lesions become inflamed, but is surprisingly rare. If the lesions become painful, rather than itchy, if they weep any purulent fluid, or if a second phase of fever develops, then a secondary infection may indeed be present. Take a swab from any weeping lesion for bacterial culture, and treat as for cellulitis (*see* page 66) to cover not only *Staphylococcus* (the common skin pathogen) but also *Streptococcus*, which has been implicated in life-threatening secondary infections following chickenpox.

Reference

• Gnann JWJ (2002) Varicella-zoster virus: atypical presentations and unusual complications. *J Infect Dis* **186** (Suppl 1): S91–8.

Urticaria

This is a rash triggered by the immune system either appropriately (infection) or inappropriately (allergy), or for an unknown reason (idiopathic).

• also called 'nettle rash'

• raised irritating wheals

• other symptoms may suggest the cause

• common causes include:

- drugs (e.g. aspirin, antibiotics)

- food allergy

- heat or sunlight

- vigorous exercise

- pressure

- cold

- viral infection

- psychosocial stress

Action
- oral (not topical) antihistamines:
  - chlorphenamine if sedation is desirable
  - loratadine or fexofenadine if sedation is not acceptable

Refer to doctor
- if drug allergy suspected, or symptoms recurrent

Scabies

- spreading variable rash
- widespread severe itching, worse at night
- rash never found on face
- sleeping partners or other family members may be affected

Action
- malathion aqueous liquid or permethrin dermal cream to all household, repeated after 7 days
- antihistamines (as above). Sedative antihistamines give the best relief from itching, but the sedation may be unacceptable
- stress that *itching may persist for several weeks* after mites have been eradicated

A rash in a seriously ill patient

A rash in a seriously ill patient may be caused by:

- measles
- meningococcal septicaemia

Measles

- rare, but increasing thanks to the MMR scare
- high fever
- cough, sometimes severe respiratory infection
- conjunctivitis
- bright red maculo-papular (flat and raised) areas which coalesce, mainly on trunk

Examination
- ears for otitis media
- chest

Action
- complete 'notification of infectious diseases' form
- refer to doctor if particularly unwell
- arrange follow-up to assess progress
- saliva tests will probably be requested later to confirm the diagnosis

Meningococcal septicaemia

- extremely rare but very important
- patient looks ill, often drowsy or confused
- fever
- diarrhoea is a common early feature
- the classic rash is purpuric (i.e. dull purplish red, does not blanch on pressure using a glass) but there may be a non-specific rash in the early stages

Refer to doctor
- *immediately* for an injection of benzyl penicillin and transfer to hospital by emergency ambulance

A rash in a mildly febrile patient

A rash in a mildly febrile patient may be caused by:

- non-specific viral infection
- parvovirus
- hand, foot and mouth disease
- streptococcal infection

Non-specific viral infection

Many viruses cause a diffuse macular rash. There are thousands of different types of virus, and the type of rash that they cause is not consistent, so it is usually impossible to name the virus. Some specific syndromes such as roseola infantum have been described, but in the absence of any specific treatment such labels are not usually helpful.

Action
- check for pharyngitis (possible streptococcal infection, *see* page 9)
- rubella is now rare, especially in children, but if an unimmunised child develops a macular rash it may be wise to inform pregnant contacts. The 'green book' is out of date on this subject: see www.hpa.org.uk/infections/topics_az/rubella/rash.pdf
- no specific treatment is available or needed for other viral infections

Refer to doctor
- if pregnant

Parvovirus

- 'slapped cheeks'
- diffuse macular rash
- cold symptoms
- joint pains in adults

Action   • no treatment needed

Refer to doctor   • if pregnant, under 30 weeks (may cause miscarriage)

Information on parvovirus in pregnancy is available at www.hpa.org.uk/infections/topics_az/rubella/rash.pdf.

Hand, foot and mouth disease

- caused by a virus
- blisters on hands, feet and in mouth
- fever and malaise
- not related to foot and mouth disease in animals

Action   • no treatment needed

Streptococcal infection

- generalised macular rash
- sore throat/exudates
- cervical lymphadenopathy
- fever and malaise

Action   • penicillin V recommended (*see* page 9)

Purple rashes

Purple rashes are usually caused by extravasation of blood from the vessels just under the skin, therefore they do not blanch on pressure or when covered by a glass (the 'tumbler test'). Pinpoint rashes are described as petechial, larger areas as purpuric. Such rashes may be caused by:

- pressure changes, e.g. attempted strangulation, violent vomiting, 'love bites'

- meningococcal septicaemia
- blood or clotting abnormalities, e.g. leukaemia, thrombocytopenia, aspirin in the elderly
- vasculitis, e.g. Henoch–Schöenlein purpura, which mainly affects children. Other features include arthritis, abdominal pain, gastrointestinal bleeding, orchitis, and nephritis

Action
- refer to doctor urgently, unless obviously due to pressure changes

Other rashes

Other rashes may be caused by:
- impetigo
- eczema
- shingles
- pityriasis rosea
- fungal infections

Impetigo

- golden crusted lesions, usually caused by *Staphylococcus*, sometimes *Streptococcus*
- commonly on faces of children, though may occur elsewhere
- may be secondary to wound or viral lesion
- patient may be systemically unwell if infection is severe

Advice
- stay off school until lesions crusted, or for 48 h after starting treatment
- use own face cloth and towel

Prescription	• topical sodium fusidate ointment if mild
	• oral flucloxacillin if severe (erythromycin or clarithromycin if the patient is allergic to penicillin)
Caution	• severe infections with cellulitis, and infections following chickenpox, may be streptococcal. Flucloxacillin is not very effective against streptococci; in these cases, add penicillin V or use co-amoxiclav
	• mupirocin should be reserved for the treatment of methicillin-resistant *Staphylococcus aureus* (MRSA).

Reference

• Public Health Laboratory Service (PHLS) (2002) *Management of Infection: guidance for primary care.* www.hpa.org.uk

Eczema

History	• duration
	• previous episodes
	• occupation
	• suspected cause (e.g. solvents, nickel, detergents, latex)
	• itch
	• discharge
	• what treatment has been tried
	• distribution
Examination	• look at offending area
	• is it infected/inflamed/weeping?
Tests	• swab if discharging
	• scrapings for fungus (if diagnosis in doubt, or treatment unsuccessful)

Action	• avoid detergents (e.g. bubble bath – even that marketed for babies)
	• if hands affected use cotton-lined rubber gloves for washing up
Prescription/ OTC	• emollients and bath additives, e.g. emulsifying ointment, hydrous ointment, Oilatum emollient (or consult pharmacist)
	• topical steroid creams (1% hydrocortisone initially)
	• antibiotics if infected (topical sodium fusidate or oral flucloxacillin, or erythromycin/clarithromycin if allergic to penicillin)
Refer to doctor	• if vesicles or severe infection
Caution	• fungal infection may look very similar but is usually asymmetrical
	• infection is common, usually with *Staphylococcus aureus*. This may cause a sudden flare of angry, itchy eczema or an impetigo-like rash. Use topical sodium fusidate or oral flucloxacillin (erythromycin if the patient is allergic to penicillin)
	• *Herpes simplex* may produce vesicles or chickenpox-like areas. Refer to doctor if suspected

Notes on eczema

• common

• may be general tendency (in atopic individuals), or localised (in response to insult to skin). It may be referred to as 'dermatitis'

• dry, cracking, sore

• cure is impossible except in acute, short-lived cases: dietary changes are not usually helpful

• reducing exposure to house dust mite may help (e.g. anti-allergenic mattress and pillow covers, wooden floors and the use of vacuum cleaners with anti-allergenic filters)

• control is the aim, using frequent (four times daily) application of emollients (e.g. emulsifying ointment) to rehydrate the skin and prevent evaporation from the surface

Caution
- topical steroids stronger than hydrocortisone may cause atrophy and thinning of the skin after prolonged use. Tiny blood vessels become visible, for which no treatment is available. The skin of the face is the most sensitive, the palms and soles least sensitive. Children's skin is more sensitive than adults' – **do not use anything stronger than hydrocortisone in children, or on the face**

- 1% hydrocortisone can be bought OTC for considerably less than the prescription charge, but the packs carry warnings not to use the product in children or on the face, and the pharmacist is not allowed to sell them for these purposes. If the patient has been assessed by a clinician, these warnings are unnecessary

A list of treatments for eczema with their steroid potencies is given in Figure 4.1.

Preparation	Steroid potency
Betamethasone	High
Clobetasone	Moderate
Hydrocortisone	Low
Emollients	Zero
Bath additives	Zero

Figure 4.1 Creams and ointments for eczema.

Reference

- DTB (2003) Topical steroids for atopic dermatitis in primary care. *Drug Ther Bull* **41**: 5–8.

Nappy rash

History
- duration
- creams tried

Examination
- mild/severe
- satellite spots
- involving skin creases

Tests	• none
Action	• frequent nappy changes
	• leave nappy off when possible
	• avoid plastic pants
	• if using washable nappies, care in sterilising/rinsing, and consider using disposable nappies temporarily
	• reassure parent that some children are simply prone to nappy rash
Prescription	• fungal superinfection is common in nappy rash. The presence of satellite spots and the involvement of the skin creases make this more likely – use clotrimazole cream for 2–3 weeks
	• if severe, use miconazole/hydrocortisone ointment for the first week
Refer to doctor or health visitor	• if not responding to treatment

Fungal infections

- of the foot (athlete's foot)
- of the flexures
- of the body ('ringworm')

History	• itchy rash, slowly spreading
	• not usually symmetrical
	• treatments previously tried
Examination	• eczema-like patches
	• often a scaly, inflamed edge
	• central area may appear normal
	• in toe webs, under breasts

Handwritten note in left margin: ✱ Fungal nail infections – usually no treatment until nail clippings sent to my surgery lab in any instance would need to see Dr so unable (onychomycosis) to give any treatment.

Action	• explain that it is an infection acquired from other humans or animals
	• keep as dry as possible
Prescription/OTC	• clotrimazole cream for 3 weeks
	• if clotrimazole or miconazole already tried, use terbinafine for one week
Refer to doctor	• if rash persists despite an adequate course of treatment

Reference

• Crawford F, Hart R, Bell-Syer S *et al.* (2000) Topical treatments for fungal infections of the skin and nails of the foot (Cochrane Review). *The Cochrane Library, Issue 2, 2000.* Update Software, Oxford.

Cold sores

History	• often recurrent on same site
	• tingling in skin before appearance of the sore
	• current or preceding febrile illness
	• exposure to strong sunlight
	• stress or other psychological trigger
Examination	• itchy, sore cluster of small blisters on a red patch, most commonly on the lips, but may be on the face, inside the mouth, or sometimes on genitalia
Tests	• none
Action	• aciclovir cream if within 48 h of appearance (not in pregnancy)
	• advise those working with babies under 6 months that they should not work until the sore has healed (*Herpes simplex* can cause a very serious illness in small babies)
	• take care not to touch eyes after touching cold sore

Refer to doctor   • if recurrent

Caution   • secondary bacterial infection of cold sore, causing yellow crusting and cellulitis (*see* Impetigo, page 54)

                    • beware of the very rare eczema herpeticum, a widespread eruption in a person with atopic eczema; can be life-threatening

Reference

• Worrell G (1991) Topical acyclovir for recurrent herpes labialis in primary care. *Can Fam Phys* **37**: 92–8.

Genital herpes

History   • intensely painful ulcers or blisters on the genitalia

                    • may be recurrent

Refer to doctor   • always; referral to genitourinary clinic may be necessary

Shingles

History   • discomfort or pain, often starts up to five days before the rash

                    • affects the area of skin supplied by one nerve root (*see* Figure 4.2)

                    • therefore only one side of the body is affected

                    • malaise, mild fever

                    • may start after a period of debility or psychosocial stress

                    • immunocompromised

                    • previous history of chickenpox

                    • commoner and more likely to cause long-term pain in those over 60 years

                    • recently becoming more common in children

Examination
- painful blisters in the area of skin supplied by one nerve root (dermatome)
- some may weep fluid (which is infectious)
- note which nerve root is affected (*see* Figure 4.2)
- if the face is affected, does the rash involve the forehead, cheek or the tip of the nose? Is the eye red?
- local lymph nodes may be enlarged

Tests
- none

Action
- explain the diagnosis:
  - the rash will dry within 1 week but may take several weeks to resolve completely
- advise:
  - keep the rash dry
  - avoid contact with newborn infants, pregnant women or people who are ill or infirm
  - a patient with chickenpox or shingles may infect someone else with chickenpox, but not with shingles. However the risk of infection is very low if the rash is covered, and routine exclusion from school and work is not necessary for patients with shingles
  - creams and lotions are of little or no help, and best avoided because of the risk of spreading skin bacteria into the blistered area
  - seek medical advice again if the rash 'flares up' (because of secondary infection)
  - malaise may require rest and time off work
- paracetamol, ibuprofen and/or dihydrocodeine for initial pain

Refer to doctor
- if aged over 60 and within 72 h of onset, to consider antiviral treatment
- if face or eye affected (*see* above)
- immunocompromised patients

- if the pain is troublesome despite simple analgesia (may need drugs for neuropathic pain)

Reference

- DTB (1998) Update on drugs for herpes zoster and genital herpes. *Drug Ther Bull* **36**: 77–9.

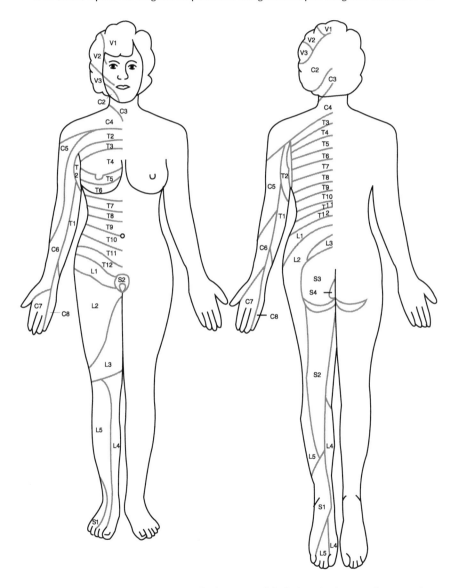

Figure 4.2 Dermatome diagram. Each area is labelled with the spinal nerve that carries sensation from the skin to the spinal cord. The areas overlap to some extent, and an individual person may vary from normal. C, cervical; L, lumbar; S, sacral; T, thoracic; V, fifth cranial nerve (trigeminal).

Pityriasis rosea

History
- an acute eruption of numerous, widespread, pink, scaly, oval patches 1–4 cm in diameter, occurring over a period of days
- usually a larger initial 'herald' patch
- the patches often follow the skin creases and mainly affect the trunk, face, scalp and upper limbs
- there may be itching, usually mild but occasionally intense
- it occurs mainly in adolescents and young adults, and more often during autumn or spring
- there may have been malaise, fever or lymphadenopathy before the rash appeared

Tests
- none

Action
- no treatment is required
- the rash will last 6–10 weeks then disappear, leaving no trace
- explain the condition and its course to the patient and reassure that it is not contagious, nor does it recur

Warts and verrucae

Examination
- raised pale bumps, or flattened areas with black dots

Explain
- caused by a virus
- most disappear by themselves with time, but may take 2–3 years
- contagious

Action
There is little evidence to prefer one treatment above another. Anecdotally, the application of a banana skin, with the white inside part taped against the wart, each night for

two weeks has often been reported to be effective – but it seems highly unlikely that a clinical trial on this treatment would ever be funded. It does have the advantage of being virtually free, with no known side-effects. Of the conventional treatments, salicylic acid appears to be the best from the limited evidence available.

Options:
1 leave alone

2 soak in warm water for 5 minutes twice daily, remove dead skin with an emery board, then apply salicylic acid. Persevere until completely disappeared; may take 3 months

3 liquid nitrogen – not for children under the age of 10 years, as can be painful. Can also cause dramatic blood blistering, temporary numbness and a scar

Even vigorous procedures do not always succeed, and warts often reappear at the treated site. A patient with a verruca should use a waterproof plaster or verruca sock for swimming and PE, and avoid sharing a towel.

Refer to doctor
• anogenital warts

• single warts in the elderly (may be a squamous carcinoma)

Reference

• Gibbs S, Harvey I, Sterling JC and Stark R (2003) Local treatments for cutaneous warts (Cochrane Review). *The Cochrane Library, Issue 3, 2003.* Update Software, Oxford.

Molluscum contagiosum

Molluscum contagiosum is a pox virus infection which produces clusters of round, raised, pearly white lesions (sometimes with a darker central dimple) on the trunk and limbs of children. It is best left untreated as it resolves completely, without scarring, after several months.

Boils

History
• duration

• fever

- thirst/polyuria/tiredness
- immunocompromised

Examination
- cellulitis
- enlarged lymph nodes
- pallor

Tests
- if recurrent boils, or symptoms or family history of diabetes, test urine for glucose (*see* Box 4.1)

Action
- apply heat to encourage pointing
- magnesium sulphate paste is traditionally used, although there is no evidence to support it
- if severe pain:
  - flucloxacillin for 7 days
  - erythromycin or clarithromycin if the patient is allergic to penicillin

Refer to doctor
- urgently if facial boil causing cellulitis (can be life-threatening), or boil in anogenital area or natal cleft (between buttocks)
- make appointment if recurrent boils

Box 4.1   Screening for diabetes

Much has been written about this, and there will be a protocol for your area based on the international criteria for the diagnosis and the characteristics of the various tests for diabetes. The protocol might start with a fasting blood glucose level as the first step, but screening whole populations in this way is burdensome and not as effective as targeting those at higher risk of diabetes. But how do you decide who is at high risk?

- *High risk:* if you strongly suspect diabetes because of classic symptoms, such as thirst, polyuria and weight loss, then formal testing with fasting blood glucose and, if necessary, a glucose tolerance test is needed. Follow your protocol.

continued overleaf

- *Moderate risk*: if the patient is at high risk of having diabetes, but has no symptoms, it is also appropriate to follow the usual protocol. For a list of risk factors see www.diabetes.org.uk/good_practice/earlyid/criteria.htm.
- *Low risk*: if the patient has a minor illness known to be more common in those with diabetes, such as cystitis or boils, but has no symptoms of diabetes, then test the urine for glucose. If this proves positive, then it is quite likely that the patient does indeed have diabetes, but this needs confirming with blood tests. If the urine is negative for glucose, this does not completely exclude diabetes (the elderly in particular may not show glucose in the urine despite fairly high blood levels), but the test is adequate when the chance of finding diabetes is low.

Testing the urine for glucose is useful in primary care when the individual's risk of diabetes is low. The test is quick, inexpensive, does not require the patient to fast, and the result is known immediately. Positive results need further investigation to establish the diagnosis.

Reference
- Davies MJ, Ammari F, Sherriff C *et al.* (1999) Screening for type 2 diabetes mellitus in the UK Indo-Asian population. *Diabet Med* **16**: 131–7.

Infected wounds/cellulitis

History
- duration
- nature of wound
- fever/malaise
- tetanus status
- immunocompromised

Examination
- discharge
- cellulitis
- lymphadenopathy

Tests
- take swabs if discharge from a significant wound

- if history of recurrent skin infections, or symptoms or family history of diabetes, test urine for glucose (*see* Box 4.1)

Action
- wound cleaning and dressing as appropriate
- sodium fusidate ointment for mild superficial infections
- oral flucloxacillin for 7 days for more severe infections (erythromycin if the patient is allergic to penicillin)
- if deeper cellulitis is present, add penicillin V to flucloxacillin, or use co-amoxiclav (erythromycin or clarithromycin if the patient is allergic to penicillin)
- consider tetanus booster

Refer to doctor
- same day if:
  - immunocompromised
  - diabetes
  - severe infection
  - pointing abscess (for incision and drainage)
  - in anogenital area or natal cleft (between buttocks)

Ingrowing toenail

History
- duration
- discharge
- previous episodes
- diabetes

Examination
- cellulitis
- discharge
- granulation

Tests	• swab if discharge
Action	• advise to insert a pledget of cotton wool or Jelonet after bathing, to lift the corner of nail away from the flesh
	• chiropody referral if persistent/recurrent
	• if localised cellulitis, give flucloxacillin for 7 days (or erythromycin/clarithromycin if allergic to penicillin)
Refer to doctor	• patients with diabetes

References

• Ingrowing toenail treatments (1999) *Bandolier* **69**: 1–2.
• Connolly B and Fitzgerald R (1988) Pledgets in ingrowing toenails. *Arch Dis Child* **63**: 71–2.

Head lice

History	• nits
	• lice
	• scratching
Examination	• examine head
	• may have enlarged lymph nodes at back of neck
	• nits (louse eggs adhere to hair tightly, whereas dandruff falls off easily)
Tests	• none
Action	• follow current local recommendations – if none, use *aqueous* malathion
	• check all of household and treat *affected people only* (repeat after 2 weeks)
	• apply conditioner liberally, then use fine metal comb to break the legs of the lice, so that they cannot reproduce.

'Bugbusting' kits are available on prescription. Although doubt has been cast on the efficacy of wet combing, many of the trials which compared this treatment with insecticides were not recent or UK based

- reassure – lice prefer clean hair

- warn patient that eggs will be visible after treatment

Refer to doctor • if recurrent problems
or health visitor

Caution • those with asthma should use *aqueous* lotions and avoid alcoholic lotions, which can cause wheezing

Reference

- Dodd CS (2001) Interventions for treating headlice (Cochrane Review). *The Cochrane Library, Issue 2, 2001.* Update Software, Oxford.

Moles

Most moles develop in early childhood and adolescence, and there is a gradual decrease in their number in old age. Not unreasonably, malignant melanoma is a concern behind many consultations, in which most patients need reassurance.

History • patient's concern about the mole

- ask about the features below

Examination There are seven points to look for and ask about:

1 size: most benign moles are less than 1 cm in diameter. Ask about any increase

2 shape: has it a regular, well-defined edge?

3 colour: is the colour even throughout, any change?

4 itching

5 spontaneous bleeding (bleeding after trauma is not a sign of malignancy)

6 crusting

7 inflammation

Tests
- none

Action
- reassure if two or fewer of the above seven points are true, in which case the mole is almost certainly not a malignant melanoma
- advise:
  - on the points above
  - to watch the mole themselves; maybe measure it or trace its outline, and come back if it is enlarging
  - to take a sensible approach to sun exposure

Refer to doctor
- if:
  - more than two of the above seven points are true
  - any mole has been increasing in size and is now over 0.5 cm in diameter
  - any change in shape or colour

Caution
- many so-called moles are, in fact, seborrhoeic keratoses (senile warts), which are superficial, golden brown in colour with a scaly, greasy surface. They are harmless
- beware slowly growing, ulcerated or raised areas with a raised edge. They may be skin carcinomas: basal cell carcinomas (rodent ulcers) are commonly found on the faces and foreheads of elderly people

Reference

- Mackie R, Doherty V, Keefe M *et al.* (1991) Seven-point checklist for melanoma. *Clin Exp Dermatol* **16**: 151–3.

Insect bites and stings

History
- site
- nature of insect, if known. You may recognise a local pattern, e.g. Blandford fly (found in an arc running from East Anglia through Oxfordshire into Dorset) which causes painful blistering or haemorrhagic lesions on the legs
- previous severe reaction to bites (suggests allergy)

Examination
- size of reaction
- is sting still *in situ* (rare)?

Tests
- none

Action
- oral antihistamine, e.g. loratadine
- avoid topical antihistamines, which are not effective and may themselves cause irritation
- anecdotally, witch hazel and aloe vera products are often reported to be soothing
- piezo-electric devices (e.g. Zanza-click) are available from pharmacies for around £7

Refer to doctor
- urgently if:
  - swelling of lips or tongue
  - anaphylactic shock (extremely rare)

Caution
- it may sometimes be difficult to distinguish allergy from infection, which usually develops after 24 h and becomes progressively worse
- recurrent bites on the legs are usually due to dog or cat fleas in carpets or rugs

Sunburn

History	• duration of exposure
	• sunscreens
Examination	• extent of burn
	• blistering
Tests	• none
Action	• safe sun advice
	• leave blisters intact if possible

There is little evidence to inform practice. Silver sulphadiazine is widely used, despite limited evidence that it may delay healing.

Mouth problems

Oral candidiasis (thrush)

A fungal infection, common in babies, those using inhaled corticosteroids and the immunocompromised.

History	• soreness
	• difficulty in eating/drinking
	• immunocompromised
Examination	• white patches on tongue and oral mucosa that cannot easily be removed
Tests	• mouth swab may be useful if the diagnosis is in doubt
Action/ prescription	• nystatin oral suspension or miconazole oral gel (OTC). There is little evidence available to compare these preparations, but nystatin is available only on prescription

- for those using inhaled steroids, ensure that spacer (e.g. Aerochamber) is used, and recommend that after use they gargle with water and then spit it out

Refer to doctor • if patient does not fall into the groups described above – this may be the first presentation of an immune deficiency

Aphthous ulcers

History • painful ulcers

• may occur anywhere in the mouth, most commonly on the buccal mucosa (lining of the cheek)

Examination • red, round lesions, sometimes with white crater

Action/ prescription • chlorhexidine oral spray (OTC)

Refer to doctor • if persisting/enlarging ulcer (may be a carcinoma)

Hand, foot and mouth disease

See page 53.

Herpes simplex stomatitis

As well as the familiar cold sore (*see* page 59), the *Herpes simplex* virus may cause a systemic illness with extensive ulceration of the mouth when it is first encountered.

History • usually a small child

• short history of fever and malaise

• refusing to eat or drink

Examination • dehydration

               • multiple small ulcers on tongue, palate and buccal mucosa (cheek lining)

Action   • ensure adequate fluid intake (a straw, or very cold drinks may help)

Refer to doctor • urgently if symptoms of less than 48 h duration, for consideration of oral aciclovir

Reference

• Amir J, Harel L, Smetana Z *et al.* (1997) Treatment of *herpes simplex* gingivostomatitis with aciclovir in children: a randomised double-blind placebo controlled study. *BMJ* **314**: 1800–3.

Dental infections

History   • site of pain

               • swelling

               • fever

               • duration

               • when dentist last consulted

Examination   • record site of pain/swelling

               • obvious dental decay

Action   • advise seeing dentist within 1 week

               • discuss analgesics

               • prescribe antibiotics (if appropriate in your place of work)

Prescription   • metronidazole for 5 days (amoxicillin if the patient is sensitive to metronidazole)

               • treatment with an appropriate antibiotic usually provides rapid relief of pain, but if additional analgesia is required suggest ibuprofen or paracetamol. Codeine can also be used, but it may be ineffective or cause an exacerbation of dental pain in some men

Reference

• Seymour RA, Rawlins MD and Rowell FJ (1982) Dihydrocodeine-induced hyperalgesia in postoperative dental pain. *Lancet* **1**: 1425–6.

5 Abdomen

Abdominal pain

History

- site
- duration
- intermittent/continuous
- stabbing/dull/colicky
- previous episodes (diagnosis and outcome)
- previous abdominal operations
- date of last menstrual period (LMP)/vaginal discharge or bleeding/contraception
- associated features:
  - fever
  - constipation/diarrhoea/blood or mucus in stool
  - vomiting/nausea/anorexia
  - dysuria/frequency
  - pain in testicles or groin
  - upper respiratory tract infection in children (may cause abdominal pain due to enlarged lymph nodes)
- OTC preparations tried

Examination

- examine abdomen, check groins for swelling
- record site of pain, any tenderness
- examine tonsils in children

Tests

- test urine for protein/blood/glucose/nitrites
- send MSU for culture if urinary symptoms present

Refer to doctor
- always, unless obvious gastroenteritis or urinary tract infection (UTI) (*see* those protocols)

- urgently if:
  - severe
  - less than 1 week history
  - testicular pain or groin swelling
  - patient is pregnant

Caution
- *Ectopic pregnancy* causes severe lower abdominal pain, usually one-sided, in a woman whose period is late or just due. She may collapse with the pain, particularly if a vaginal examination is attempted. If suspected, refer to doctor urgently.

Dyspepsia

History
- what does the patient mean by the words they use?
- site of pain/discomfort
- heartburn
- relation to meals
- relation to exercise
- smoking
- alcohol
- diet (e.g. irregular meals, large meals at night, fatty foods, excessive citrus fruit juices can all cause digestive symptoms)
- psychosocial stress
- associated symptoms:
  - vomiting
  - bowel habit/motion colour
  - weight loss
- previous episodes, how treated

- OTC preparations tried
- drugs, especially aspirin, non-steroidal anti-inflammatory drugs (NSAIDs), prednisolone, bisphosphonates used to treat osteoporosis

Examination
- feel abdomen
- record site of pain

Tests
- none

Action
- stop any NSAID, unless patient has rheumatoid arthritis (in which case refer to doctor)
- do not stop aspirin prescribed for ischaemic heart disease or stroke prevention – refer to prescriber
- advise antacids initially
- ranitidine if antacids have been tried and are ineffective
- advise on diet and lifestyle

Prescription/OTC
- antacids; magnesium trisilicate or Gaviscon Advance (both OTC)
- ranitidine for 7 days (available OTC for less than the prescription charge, but at lower dosage)

Refer to doctor
- urgently if:
  - sudden onset or related to exercise (may be cardiac)
  - vomiting
  - gastrointestinal bleeding
  - unintentional weight loss
  - difficulty in swallowing
- routinely if:
  - aged over 55 years
  - persistent/recurrent symptoms
  - patient is on medication that may need to be reviewed

Reference

• Chatfield S (1999) A comparison of the efficacy of the alginate preparation, Gaviscon Advance, with placebo in the treatment of gastro-oesophageal reflux disease. *Curr Med Res Opin* **15**: 152–9.

Diarrhoea and vomiting

History
- duration: preceding constipation
- severity: number of episodes in last 24 h, stool consistency
- blood (red, brown or black) in motion/vomit
- fever
- contacts with similar symptoms, especially if they started on the same day
- foreign travel
- suspect meals or foods. NB sorbitol (in diet foods, chewing gum) may cause diarrhoea in large doses
- occupation: food handler/carer/health professional
- in children: adequate urine output
- previous bowel disease
- immunocompromised
- relevant medication (e.g. antibiotics, NSAIDs, metformin, laxatives, opioids)

Examination
- dehydration:
  - fontanelle in babies under 1 year
  - dry tongue/mouth
  - dry skin not reshaping after a soft pinch
  - dry eyes, no tears, not reflecting light
- consider abdominal examination, if pain is prominent
- consider rectal examination if overflow suspected (*see* Caution)

Test

Stool culture if:

- suspicion of food poisoning
- febrile/systemically unwell
- blood in stool
- watery diarrhoea for 4 days or more
- recent broad spectrum antibiotic therapy (ask the laboratory to look for *Clostridium difficile*)
- immunocompromised
- recent travel to countries with poor hygiene
- food handler/carer working in institution/healthcare staff

(Recommended method: ask patient to collect 5 ml sample in clingfilm-lined container, avoiding touching anything that the sample will contact. Write patient's name on specimen bottle.)

- also check MSU in children under five with persistent or recurrent diarrhoea or vomiting (*see* page 86)

Action

- reassurance: rarely serious
- dehydration is rare over 6 months of age (explain warning signs)
- recommend care when washing hands after using toilet/ changing nappy
- food handlers, carers in institutions and healthcare staff should not work until free of symptoms for 48 h
- extra fluids should be taken, especially fruit juice (prefer- ably not orange juice) and soup
- fasting is no longer recommended. A normal diet should be resumed as soon as symptoms permit. High-carbohydrate foods such as boiled rice or stewed apple seem to be most beneficial
- there is some evidence that probiotics such as lacto- bacillus may be helpful, especially in diarrhoea following broad-spectrum antibiotics. These can be found in live yoghourt products such as Yakult and Actimel, or in capsules from health food shops

> **Box 5.1   Lactose intolerance**
>
> Occasionally, after a bout of gastroenteritis, small children may develop a temporary inability to digest lactose, which may delay the resolution of their diarrhoea. If this is suspected, suggest using lactose-free milk (e.g. SMA LF) for a few days only.

Prescription/OTC   (none for most patients)

- paracetamol for stomach cramps (advise avoiding ibuprofen and aspirin)

- loperamide for adults if diarrhoea is disabling. Avoid if there is blood in the stool or severe malaise

- adult patients who are very unwell or socially devastated by their symptoms could be offered buccal prochlorperazine (available OTC) for vomiting in those over 20 years

Notification

- notify immediately if food poisoning suspected because of the history, or symptom of bloody diarrhoea, or if confirmed by culture. Complete form from *Notification of Infectious Diseases* book. Tell patients that someone from the Health Protection Unit may contact them (*see* Chapter 9).

Refer to doctor

- urgently if:
  - diabetes
  - immunocompromised
  - inflammatory bowel disease (ulcerative colitis or Crohn's)
  - diverticular disease
  - symptoms are side-effects of a drug which will need to be changed (urgency of referral depends on why the drug was prescribed)
  - blood (red or brown) in vomit
  - significant blood (red or black) in stools

– severe diarrhoea and malaise, especially if recently returned from abroad, for consideration of ciprofloxacin therapy

Caution
- spurious or 'overflow' diarrhoea may be caused by severe constipation. If in doubt, do a rectal examination

- diarrhoea may be an early feature of meningococcal septicaemia

- gastrointestinal side-effects from drugs are common, especially if the patient has recently started an analgesic or an antibiotic

References

- Allen SJ, Okoko B, Martinez E *et al.* (2003) Probiotics for treating infectious diarrhoea (Cochrane Review). *The Cochrane Library, Issue 4, 2003.* Update Software, Oxford.
- Farthing M, Feldman R, Finch R *et al.* (1996) The management of infective gastroenteritis in adults. A consensus statement by an expert panel convened by the British Society for the Study of Infection. *J Infect* **33**: 143–52.
- Nutrition Committee, Canadian Pediatric Society (2002) Oral rehydration therapy and early refeeding in the management of childhood gastroenteritis. Canadian Paediatric Society, Ottawa. www.cps.ca/english/statements/N/n94–03.htm

Constipation

History
- duration; habitual

- how often bowels open

- consistency of motion/straining

- blood in stool, on toilet paper or in toilet pan

- abdominal pain

- vomiting

- previous abdominal operations

- unintentional weight loss

- medication (e.g. analgesics containing codeine, tricyclic antidepressants)

- amount of exercise

Examination	• usually none
	• consider rectal examination if diagnosis/severity in doubt
Tests	• none
Action	• high-fibre diet
	• high fluid intake (two litres per day)
	• increase exercise
	• review drugs, especially codeine preparations
	• ispaghula husk may be used, if fibre intake is insufficient
	• senna is quick acting, but may cause abdominal cramps
	• treatment may need to continue for several weeks
	• glycerol suppositories give the fastest relief in distal constipation
Refer to doctor	• urgently if:
	– associated with vomiting and/or previous abdominal surgery
	• routinely if:
	– sudden change in bowel habit, unintentional weight loss or rectal bleeding in adults
	– symptoms persist

Rectal problems

> ## Box 5.2 Rectal problems
>
> ### Haemorrhoids ('piles')
>
> These are distended veins inside the anal canal, which have a similar appearance to varicose veins. They may prolapse ('come down') on straining, when they may be visible as soft, purple grape-like swellings protruding from the anus. They may cause bleeding, itching or discomfort.
>
> ### Thrombosed external pile
>
> This is caused by a sudden leakage of blood from a small blood vessel near the anus. The blood stretches the sensitive skin and is very painful. It will gradually disperse, but if the patient presents early it is possible to incise it and relieve pain by releasing the blood clot.
>
> ### Anal fissure
>
> A split in the anal skin, thought to be caused by passing a large, hard stool. This is a common cause of pain and bleeding on defaecation. Most will heal within 6 weeks, provided that the stools remain soft.

History
- bleeding on defaecation:
  - how much, in toilet pan/on paper only?
  - bright red/dark red
- pain on defaecation
- itch (threadworms)
- swelling near anus, or does a swelling appear on straining?
- constipation

Examination   (may be normal if haemorrhoids are internal)
- any visible swelling

- any split in peri-anal skin
- worms may be seen

Action
- advise:
  - avoid straining
  - high-fibre diet
  - drink 2 l of fluid daily
  - warm baths may be soothing
  - alternate wet /dry toilet tissue
  - if the pain of thrombosed piles is severe, relief may be obtained by sitting on something cold

Prescription/OTC
- consider ispaghula husk short term
- Anusol cream, or Xyloproct if pain is severe

Refer to doctor
- urgently if:
  - severe bleeding
  - dark blood (may come from a carcinoma high inside the bowel)
- routinely if:
  - persistent or recurrent problems

Caution
- remember the possibility of sexual abuse or sexually transmitted diseases
- threadworms are the commonest cause of anal discomfort in children

Urinary tract infection/cystitis

History
- duration
- dysuria/frequency

- obvious haematuria

- fever/abdominal pain/vomiting

- loin pain

- vaginal discharge

- recurrent symptoms

- associated with intercourse (NB teenagers may need contraception)

- possibility of pregnancy

- previous history of renal stones or pyelonephritis

Examination
- in small boys check the penis for redness (*see* balanitis, page 90)

Tests
- urinalysis for blood/protein, nitrites, if urine readily available (to avoid contaminating the whole sample, pour a little urine on to the test strip). A positive nitrite test is diagnostic, but a negative test does not exclude infection

- an MSU is essential before starting treatment in:

  - children. Bag or pad samples may be needed in infants. Older children should be encouraged to pass a sample directly into a sterile container, but if this proves impossible it is reasonable to collect a sample from a clingfilm-lined container or potty

  - men

  - pregnant women

  - those with persistent recurrent symptoms

  - those with fever/loin pain

- an MSU may be helpful in all cases, to identify culture negative cystitis (*Chlamydia*?) and to identify treatment failures

- arrange follow-up MSU after treatment (unnecessary for uncomplicated UTI in women)

- if associated vaginal discharge

- high vaginal and cervical swabs for culture and *Chlamydia* test

Action
- ensure adequate fluid intake
- OTC remedies such as Cymalon or Cystemme make the urine more alkaline, and are said to relieve the discomfort of cystitis. There is little evidence to support their use
- cranberry juice has previously been recommended, but a systematic review found no evidence that it reduced the symptoms of an acute attack. It should not be taken by patients on anticoagulants
- ask patient to phone for MSU results (if applicable)

Prescription
- antibiotics:
  - uncomplicated UTI in non-pregnant women: trimethoprim for 3 days *or* nitrofurantoin m/r (modified release) for 3 days (depending on local patterns of antibiotic resistance)
  - children or men: trimethoprim for 7 days (or cefalexin for 7 days if allergic to trimethoprim)
  - pregnant women: cefalexin for 7 days

Refer to doctor
- urgently if:
  - suspected pyelonephritis (fever/loin pain/malaise) – will need treatment with cefalexin for 14 days and possible referral)
  - history of kidney stones/pyelonephritis
- routinely (when UTI confirmed by MSU result) in:
  - children (*important*: urine infections in small children may cause permanent kidney damage)
  - men (for assessment of prostate and possible further investigation)
  - women with severe/persistent symptoms

Caution
- in children and pregnant women, do not wait for the MSU result before starting antibiotics. (UTI in early pregnancy increases the risk of miscarriage)
- women sometimes confuse the symptoms of thrush and cystitis
- *Chlamydia* infections may cause dysuria

References

- DTB (1997) The management of urinary tract infection in children. *Drug Ther Bull* **35**: 65–9.
- DTB (2005) Cranberry and urinary tract infection. *Drug Ther Bull* **43**: 17–19.
- Brumfitt W, Hamilton-Miller JM, Cooper J *et al.* (1990) Relationship of urinary pH to symptoms of 'cystitis'. *Postgrad Med J* **66**: 727–9.

Threadworms

History
- peri-anal irritation
- anal discomfort at night
- worms may be seen – like white cotton threads – on skin or in stool

Examination
- not necessary

Test

Tests are not necessary unless the diagnosis is in doubt. Sellotape applied to the anus first thing in the morning will pick up the eggs. Stick the Sellotape on to a microscope slide labelled with the patient's name and send it to the laboratory for confirmation of the diagnosis.

Action
- an appointment is not necessary if the parent is sure of the diagnosis
- explain that adult threadworms live for only six weeks – their eggs must be transferred to the mouth and swallowed for the infection to continue
- as well as the prescription, hygienic measures are necessary:
  - wash hands and scrub nails before each meal and after going to the toilet
  - bathe or shower in early morning to remove eggs laid during the night
  - wear close-fitting pants in bed
  - change bed linen, underwear and night clothes frequently
  - vacuum bedroom carpet frequently
  - cut fingernails short

Treatment	• mebendazole for adults (unless pregnant or breast-feeding) and children over 2 years. A second dose may be needed two weeks later
	• piperazine/senna for children under 2 years and infection in lactating women
	• treat all members of household simultaneously
Refer to doctor	• if pregnant – treatment is controversial

Reference

Anon (1999) Threadworms. *Presc Nurse Bull* **1**: 11–12.

Balanitis (sore penis)

History	• duration
	• swelling of foreskin
	• discharge
	• dysuria
	• previous episodes
	• diabetes
	• immunocompromised
Examination	• gently attempt to retract foreskin in boys aged 3 years and over
	• localised redness/generalised cellulitis
Tests	• take swab, if discharge
	• send MSU for culture if no redness visible
	• consider testing urine for glucose in adults
Action	• advise gentle cleaning under foreskin in boys aged 3 years and over (ensure it is pulled down afterwards)
	• if difficulty in passing urine because of pain, sit in bath

Prescription
- clotrimazole cream in adults
- sodium fusidate ointment for mild infections in children
- co-amoxiclav for 7 days if cellulitis present in a child (erythromycin if allergic to penicillin)

Refer to doctor
- urgently, if:
  - immunocompromised
  - severe symptoms or swab negative in adults (may need referral to genitourinary clinic)
- routinely, if:
  - recurrent episodes in children (may need surgical treatment)

Caution
- if no visible redness, this may be a UTI
- Candida is the commonest cause of balanitis in adults. Very little research is available to guide practice on balanitis in children

References

- Clinical Effectiveness Group (1999) National guideline for the management of balanitis. *Sex Transm Infect* **75** (Suppl 1): S85–S88. www.bashh.org
- Schwartz RH (1996) Acute balanoposthitis in young boys. *Paed Inf Dis* **15**: 176–7.

6 Women's health

Vaginal discharge

History
- duration
- colour
- smell – if offensive, possible retained tampon
- itch
- abdominal pain
- fever
- irregular bleeding
- previous episodes
- timing with menstrual cycle
- recent broad-spectrum antibiotics
- pregnant
- immunocompromised

Examination
- not necessary if symptoms typical of candidal infection which has been previously diagnosed by culture and successfully treated
- may be needed to check for retained tampon
- look for 'cottage cheese' appearance of thrush

Tests
- high vaginal swab (HVS)
- consider also cervical swabs for bacterial and chlamydial tests if diagnosis not obvious
- if recurrent or severe thrush, check urine for glucose

Action
- if thrush:
  - clotrimazole pessary or oral fluconazole (equally effective, and now only slightly more expensive)

- maybe also clotrimazole cream if signs of external thrush, or miconazole/hydrocortisone ointment if itching severe

- no need to treat male partner, unless he has symptoms

- if recurrent, suggest cotton pants, and avoid tights, bubble bath and biological washing powders. There is no evidence to support the use of live yoghourt

- if pregnant, clotrimazole is regarded as safe but longer courses may be needed, e.g. 100 mg pessary for six nights

- if diagnosis uncertain, wait for HVS result. If bacterial vaginosis found (report may say 'clue cells seen') give metronidazole for 5 days and advise patient to avoid douching

Refer to doctor
- same day if:

  - abdominal pain

  - fever

  - genital blisters

- routinely if:

  - recurrent symptoms

Caution
- genital herpes – symptoms:

  - blisters

  - pain rather than itch

- pelvic inflammatory disease – symptoms:

  - abdominal pain

  - fever

  - irregular bleeding

References

- Watson MC, Grimshaw JM, Bond CM *et al.* (2002) Oral versus intra-vaginal imidazole and triazole anti-fungal agents for the treatment of uncomplicated vulvovaginal candidiasis (thrush): a systematic review. *BJOG* **109**: 85–95.
- Young GL and Jewell D (2001) Topical treatment for vaginal candidiasis (thrush) in pregnancy (Cochrane Review). *The Cochrane Library, Issue 3, 2001.* Update Software, Oxford.

Menorrhagia (heavy periods)

History	• duration and heaviness of this period
	• usual pattern of menstrual cycle
	• clots/flooding
	• pain
	• previous episodes
	• whether intrauterine contraceptive device (IUCD) fitted
	• was this period late (possibility of miscarriage)
	• hot flushes/sweats (if aged over 40 years)
Examination	• not necessary urgently
Tests	• FBC and ferritin
Action	• reassure patient there is no link between 'clots' and 'thrombosis'
	• consider recommending ferrous sulphate if iron deficient
	• ibuprofen often significantly reduces menstrual flow. It is chemically related to mefenamic acid (Ponstan) but has a better side-effect profile
	• if the above fails, norethisterone for 10 days will stop the bleeding within two or three days. A light period will occur after stopping tablets
Refer to doctor	• always, for vaginal examination and discussion of treatment options, once bleeding has stopped
	• post-menopausal bleeding (after six months of amenorrhoea) should be investigated
Caution	• miscarriage

Reference

• Makarainen L and Ylikorkala O (1986) Primary and myoma-associated menorrhagia: role of prostaglandin and effects of ibuprofen. *BJOG* **93**: 974–8.

Missed pills

History
- type of pill: combined; progestogen-only; Cerazette?
- how far into this packet?
- how many missed pills?
- how late?
- unprotected sexual intercourse (UPSI) in last two weeks?

Examination
- none

Tests
- none

Action
- advise the patient to take the last missed pill now, then resume normal pill-taking

  also:

- **if on combined oral contraceptive**, and missed two active pills or more of 20 mcg COC, or three active pills or more of 30 mcg COC:

  - for the next seven days advise using condoms or avoiding penetrative sex

  - if there are less than seven pills left in the pack, advise omit the pill-free week (or placebo tablets for ED (every day) pills). This may cause unexpected bleeding, especially with phasic pills

  - if pill-free interval has been extended and UPSI since end of last pack, consider emergency contraception (*see* pages 98–101)

Reference
- Faculty of Family Planning and Reproductive Health Care Clinical Effectiveness Unit (2005) *Missed pills: new recommendations.* www.ffprhc.org.uk/admin/uploads/MissedPillRules%20.pdf (accessed 4 August 2005).

- **if on progestogen-only contraceptive**, and 3 or more hours late (12 h for Cerazette):

  - if UPSI has occurred since the last pill was taken, consider emergency contraception (*see* pages 98–101)

– contraceptive protection will be lost. For the next 48 h use a condom also, or do not have penetrative sex

If the problem is complex you, or the patient, can ring the Family Planning Association (FPA) helpline for advice on +44 (0)845 310 1334 (9:00 to 18:00 Monday to Friday).

Reference

- Guillebaud J (2003) *Contraception, Your Questions Answered.* Churchill Livingstone, Edinburgh.

Intermenstrual bleeding

History	• menstrual cycle/date of last menstrual period (LMP)
	• previous episodes
	• fever
	• abdominal pain
	• offensive discharge
	• first experience of penetrative sex
	• any possibility of pregnancy
	• contraceptive method (if on oral contraceptive, missed pills/vomiting/antibiotics)
	• taking hormone replacement therapy (HRT)
	• missed pills
Examination	• not necessary urgently unless pain/fever/discharge present, in which case refer
Tests	• consider pregnancy test
Action	• if missed contraceptive pills/vomiting/antibiotic: *see* missed pill advice (page 96)
	• if first experience of penetrative sex, reassure that some bleeding is common

- if missed HRT tablets, resume tablet taking and make appointment if bleeding persists

- otherwise, make appointment with doctor for vaginal examination when bleeding stops

Refer to doctor
- immediately if:
  - abdominal pain/fever/offensive discharge (could be pelvic inflammatory disease)
  - pregnant
- routinely if no obvious cause for symptom

Caution
- very rarely, carcinoma of cervix/uterus/ovary may present in this way

Emergency contraception (EC)

Emergency oral contraception

History
- if under 16, check if Fraser competent (previously Gillick competent – *see* Box 6.1)
- date of LMP
  - time since UPSI (must be 72 h or less)
- previous UPSI this cycle (may render treatment in-effective – consider IUCD)
- contraceptive method: missed pills, late injection
- previous emergency contraception this cycle
- on enzyme-inducing medication, e.g. carbamazepine, phenytoin, rifampicin, terbinafine, long-term fluconazole
- taking St John's wort
- breastfeeding
- past history of porphyria (contraindicated)

consensual. 'when.
(72hrs/less)

LMP

Normal Cont.

Prev emerg cont This
cycle

15.38

Para / left wrist

since Friday.

R handed

No injury

~~Flex~~.

Carpal tunnel
to left hand

Swelling

although

No bruising

not bothering
at the
moment

Finkelstein~~s~~

~~Dequavaines~~
? Tenosinoritis

Tendonitis

Tests	• none

Action	Advise:

- may cause nausea
- seek help if vomiting occurs within 3 h of taking tablet
- use condoms, or do not have penetrative sex, until next period, which may be early or late
- explain failure rate: if 500 women take EC within 24 h of UPSI, one will become pregnant. The risk is highest at midcycle
- advise pregnancy test if next period more than 1 week late, also if on COC and continuing the packet; she may experience a withdrawal bleed even if pregnant
- no known adverse effect on foetus if pregnancy occurs, but ectopic pregnancy more likely
- if lactating, no known adverse effect on baby
- discuss long-term contraception and safe sex

Prescription	• two levonorgestrel 750 μg tablets, to be taken together as soon as possible

- an emergency IUCD is the more reliable option for those on enzyme-inducing drugs, but if the woman declines this she should be offered three tablets of levonorgestrel 750 μg, to be taken together (*BNF* 48)

Refer to doctor	• if more than 72 h since UPSI (levonorgestrel still has some benefit, but not licensed)

- if pregnant

Caution	• if patient vomits within 3 h of taking either dose, give replacement prescription for two tablets, also domperidone tablets to be taken 30 minutes before levonorgestrel dose

If the problem is complex you, or the patient, can ring the Family Planning Association (FPA) helpline for advice on +44 (0)845 310 1334 (9:00 to 18:00 Monday to Friday).

Reference

* World Health Organization (1998) Randomised controlled trial of levonorgestrel versus the Yuzpe regime of combined oral contraceptives for emergency contraception. *Lancet* **352**: 428–33.

Box 6.1   Legal issues relating to providing emergency contraception to girls aged under 16 years

In the UK, people under the age of 16 years can consent to medical treatment if they have sufficient maturity and judgement to enable them to fully understand what is proposed.

In England and Wales, it is lawful to provide contraceptive advice and treatment without parental consent, provided that the practitioner is satisfied that the following Fraser Guideline criteria are met:

* the young person understands the practitioner's advice
* the young person cannot be persuaded to inform his or her parents or to allow the practitioner to inform the parents that contraceptive advice has been sought
* the young person is likely to begin or to continue having intercourse with or without contraceptive treatment. Unless he or she receives contraceptive advice or treatment, the young person's physical or mental health or both are likely to suffer
* the young person's best interest requires the practitioner to give contraceptive advice, treatment, or both without parental consent.

In Scotland, statutory provision by way of The Age of Legal Capacity Act 1991 applies similar criteria. The Act actually appears to assign more legal rights to children under 16 years, in that parental responsibility cannot authorise procedures a competent child has refused.

Note: child protection issues should be taken into account – it is important to be satisfied that sex has been consensual and is not occurring in an incestuous relationship. If it is suspected that force has been used or that any sexual abuse has occurred, healthcare professionals have a duty to follow national and local child protection procedures.

Source: PRODIGY guidance on emergency contraception, www.prodigy.nhs.uk/

Emergency IUCD contraception

History	• if under 16 years, check if Fraser competent (previously Gillick competent – *see* Box 6.1)
	• LMP
	• recent pregnancy
	• past history of:
	– pelvic inflammatory disease (in last three months)
	– ectopic pregnancy
	– operations on fallopian tubes
Examination	• will be done by clinician fitting IUCD
Tests	• cervical swab for *Chlamydia*
Action	• a copper IUCD can be fitted up to day 19 of a 28-day cycle, regardless of the date of UPSI; the factors listed above are contraindications

Mastitis (in a lactating woman)

History	• fever
	• pain
	• redness of breast
Examination	• record area of redness
	• any suggestion of an abscess
Tests	• none
Action	• advise to continue breastfeeding (unless pus from nipple)
	• offer affected breast to baby first, to ensure good drainage

Prescription   • flucloxacillin for 7 days (cefalexin if the patient is allergic to penicillin)

Refer to doctor   • if abscess formation

Reference

• Dahlbeck SW, Donnelly JF and Theriault RL (1995) Differentiating inflammatory breast cancer from acute mastitis. *Am Fam Physician* **52**: 929–34.

7 Mental health

Depression

This is a very common condition, in which physical symptoms are often presented initially. Be aware that it may be an underlying problem in any consultation.

History
- active, sympathetic listening
- how long has the patient felt low
- any special reason, e.g. bereavement, childbirth, relationship difficulties, financial worries, stress at work
- previous episodes and treatment, and what previously helped them to resolve their problems
- medication, alcohol intake, recreational drugs
- appetite or weight change
- sleep disturbance/fatigue
- feelings of worthlessness
- thoughts of death: 'Have you ever felt that life wasn't worth living?'
- loss of concentration/poor memory
- lack of enthusiasm/enjoyment: 'What are you looking forward to?'
- ask: 'How will you know when you are better? What will you be doing that you aren't doing now?'

Examination
- observe body language, especially moist eyes, trembling lower lip

Tests
- none

Actions

- empathise and be positive about recovery

- remind patient that they have already learnt coping strategies that have previously helped them

- if taking regular medication, check listed side-effects in Summary of Product Characteristics (SPC) online at http://emc.medicines.org.uk, or summary of major side-effects in the *BNF*

- consider practical, problem-solving suggestions, e.g. a change of job

- advise regular exercise, especially walking with relative or friend

- encourage them to resume activities they previously enjoyed

- discuss alcohol and advise moderation

- discuss diet – although controversial, there is some evidence that the following may help:

  - omega-3 fish oils 10 g daily

  - vitamin B complex

  - 5-hydroxytryptophan (5-HTP) 100 mg twice daily (from health food shop or online retailer)

  - wholegrain foods

- suggest relaxation techniques (depression is often driven by anxiety)

- recommend self-help books (*see* 'resources for patients' page 109)

- discuss referral to counsellor, or other form of talking therapy

- if severe, discuss antidepressants – emphasise not addictive/3 week delay before onset of action/course will last several months

- if mild or moderate, discuss St John's wort

Refer urgently to doctor or community mental health team	• if symptoms are severe or suicidal thoughts are expressed

Caution	• some drugs can cause depression
	• St John's wort interacts with many drugs, notably combined oral contraceptives, warfarin, triptan drugs (for migraine) and anticonvulsants. *See* Appendix 1 of *BNF*

References

• Alpert JE and Fava M (1997) Nutrition and depression: the role of folate. *Nutr Rev* **55**: 145–9.
• Linde K and Mulrow CD (2003) St John's Wort for depression (Cochrane Review). In: *The Cochrane Library, Issue 2, 2003*. Update Software, Oxford.
• Holford P (2003) *Optimum Nutrition for the Mind*. Piatkus, London.

Insomnia

Insomnia is common and subjective. Some people only require four or five hours' sleep a night, whereas others need 10 h or more. The amount of sleep required tends to lessen with age and also with lower activity levels. A 'good night's sleep' is not the same for everyone. Almost everyone will have periods of insomnia at some stage.

History	• what is the patient's concern about the sleeping pattern?
	• when did the problem start, and what was happening to them at that time?
	• what is the sleep pattern:
	– difficulty getting off to sleep?
	– recurrent waking during the night?
	– early morning waking feeling unrefreshed?
	• what was previous pattern like?
	• does the patient take daytime naps?
	• does their partner say that they snore and are restless?

- general health
- medication
- caffeine, nicotine, alcohol, recreational drugs
- lifestyle – e.g. shift work
- what are the patient's expectations? – explore their ideas

Consider causes:

- *physical*: pain, itching, shortness of breath, nocturia, indigestion, tinnitus, discomfort, too warm, too cold, noise, room not dark
- *physiological*: shift work, jet lag, pregnancy
- *psychological*: emotional upsets, worries, bereavement
- *psychiatric*: especially depression, hypomania
- *pathological*: sleep apnoea, restless leg syndrome
- *pharmacological*: is patient on any medication possibly causing insomnia, e.g. corticosteroids, propranolol, pseudo-ephedrine or laxatives, or taking excessive coffee, tea, cola, alcohol, or nicotine?
- *social*: new baby, shift work, enuretic child, partner who has nocturia or who snores

Examination
- look for agitation, depression, 'washed out' appearance
- note if obese (associated with sleep apnoea syndrome)

Tests
- none

Action
- deal with underlying cause, where possible

Advice
- avoid going to bed until you feel sleepy
- take a warm, milky drink before bedtime
- regular exercise is helpful, but not just before bedtime
- relaxation exercises or training (e.g. hypnotherapy) can be helpful; also yoga, t'ai chi, meditation, reading and listening to relaxing music

- avoid lying in bed unable to get to sleep – it is better to get up and do something fairly mindless but useful, e.g. ironing

- try to wake at the same time each day using an alarm clock and do not sleep on

Prescription/OTC • hypnotic drugs such as temazepam may cause addiction, daytime drowsiness and rebound insomnia on stopping. It is therefore best to avoid these drugs. If essential, give temazepam 10 mg tablets, one at night for a maximum of 10 days. Warn that they may impair driving the next morning

- OTC remedies such as Nytol may contain sedative anti-histamines (which are temporarily effective but often cause morning drowsiness) or herbs such as valerian

Refer to doctor • if psychiatric problem

- if problem is due to prescribed drugs or treatable physical cause

- if obese and reporting snoring and excessive tiredness (may need assessment for sleep apnoea syndrome)

- if there is a risk to safety (e.g. driving when tired)

Anxiety/panic attacks/phobias

History • active, sympathetic listening

- why have they come?

- problems: at work, at home, with relatives, financial

- alcohol intake

- recreational drugs

- previous problems, and how they resolved them

- ask: 'How will you know when you are better? What will you be doing that you aren't doing now?'

- ask: 'How can I help?'

Examination	• observe body language, especially tremor
Tests	• take blood for thyroid function tests, if not recently done
Actions	• empathise and be positive about recovery
	• remind patient that they have already learnt coping strategies that have previously helped them
	• consider practical, problem-solving suggestions, e.g. a change of job
	• explain limitations of drug treatment for anxiety
	• advise exercise, especially walking
	• discuss alcohol and advise moderation
	• relaxation exercises or training (e.g. hypnotherapy) can be helpful; also yoga, t'ai chi, meditation, reading and listening to relaxing music
	• recommend self-help books (*see* 'resources for patients' page 215)
	• discuss other available agencies
Refer to doctor or community health team	• if drug treatment requested or follow-up required

Hyperventilation

History	• 'unable to take a deep enough breath'
	• absence of other respiratory symptoms, e.g. cough/malaise
	• precipitating stress
	• previous episodes
	• tingling round mouth, hands, feet
	• spasm of hands and feet (tetany)

Examination
(to exclude
respiratory
disease)
	• observe respiration – often irregular or sighing, using upper chest muscles
	• listen to chest:
	   – breath sounds are equal on both sides (to exclude pneumothorax)
	   – no wheeze (asthma)
	• record peak flow (if low, *see* Asthma, page 24)

Test	• pulse oximetry, if available, may demonstrate to the patient that they are hyperventilating
Action	• explain problem • if acute, ask patient to breathe slowly in and out of paper bag, or put hands on head to splint upper chest • suggest yoga (breathing exercises and relaxation both likely to be helpful) • relaxation exercises/hypnotherapy may lower the underlying emotional arousal

Refer to doctor	• urgently if:
	   – unequal/abnormal breath sounds
	   – peak flow less than 75% of predicted value
	   – problem does not respond promptly to treatment
	• routinely if:
	   – underlying stresses need attention
	   – breathing pattern remains disturbed (may need specialist physiotherapy referral)

Resources for patients

Books/CD ROMs: see list in 'Useful resources', particularly those listed below:

• Griffin J and Tyrell I (2004) *How to Lift Depression Fast.* HG Publishing, Chalvington.
• Bishop P (2004) *Relax ... Using Your Own Innate Resources to Let Go of Pent-up Stress and Negative Emotion* (CD-ROM audiobook) HG Publishing, Chalvington. (£10 plus £2.50 delivery from +44 (0)1323 811662 or www.humangivens.com)

Agencies:
- local counsellors (or other talking therapy)
- health visitor (mainly for parents of small children)
- Relate
- Citizens' Advice Bureau (particularly helpful for debt problems)
- Samaritans (+44 (0)8457 909090)

8 Injuries

Minor injuries

History
- severity of impact (may suggest likely consequences)
- impairment of function
- relevant medical and drug history, particularly anti-coagulants

Examination
- swelling (NB this takes time to develop – in primary care patients often present very early)
- deformity
- bony tenderness
- restriction of movement

Action
- mobilise early, after 48 h rest
- ice (e.g. pack of frozen peas, wrapped in a towel to avoid skin damage)
- NSAID topically for small area soft tissue injuries (e.g. ibuprofen gel or counter-irritant Algesal), otherwise orally if tolerated
- compression may be a valuable early treatment for joint injuries, with the exception of the ankle where there is no evidence of benefit
- elevation above the level of the heart

Refer to emergency department
- if deformity
- if severe pain
- if bony tenderness
- if unable to bear weight on leg

References

- Stiell IG, Greenbergh GH, McKnight RD *et al.* (1992) A study to develop clinical rules for the use of radiography in acute ankle injuries. *Ann Emerg Med* **21**: 384–90.
- Wilson S and Cooke M (1998) Double bandaging of sprained ankles. *BMJ* **317**: 1722–3.

Head injuries

History
- how did it happen?
- loss of consciousness
- confusion, convulsions, amnesia
- vomiting
- headache, drowsiness
- neurological disturbance (e.g. numbness, paralysis, double vision)
- bleeding disorder, anticoagulants
- recent alcohol or recreational drug use

Examination
- is the patient still confused or drowsy?
- look at injury
- check pupils:
  - are they equal?
  - do they react to light?
  - photophobia?

Tests
- none

Action
- give head injury instructions, if minor injury (*see* Box 8.1)

Refer to doctor
- high-energy impact to head
- loss of consciousness or amnesia
- confusion
- convulsions

- vomiting (more than once)
- suspected skull fracture (orbital haematoma, deafness, clear cerebrospinal fluid from ear or nose)
- substance intoxication
- neurological disturbance
- unequal pupils
- bleeding disorder or on anticoagulants
- no-one to supervise patient at home
- age >65 years (National Institute for Clinical Excellence (NICE) guidance)

Box 8.1   Head injury instructions (based on NICE guidance 2003, adapted for primary care)

Any injury or blow to the head will cause a certain degree of concussion. The seriousness of the concussion depends upon the severity of the injury. Nearly all patients with even slight concussion will probably have a headache for 48 h. They may well feel a little washed out and irritable during this period. Children often feel sick and may vomit and appear to be sleepy. This is to be expected in children who have had a blow to the head, and lasts 12–24 h.

Should

- the headache become severe
- the vomiting increase
- the sleepiness increase so that it is difficult to get the person to talk
- the irritability increase
- the person find that bright light in the eyes causes distress
- the person have a fit

then the person should be taken immediately to hospital for a further examination.

An adult with a suspected head injury should not return home alone.

A child with a head injury should not be left unattended at home for any length of time.

Simple paracetamol is suitable for pain relief.

continued overleaf

Advice to an adult after a head injury

- rest as much as possible, take a few days off work or study
- take paracetamol for headache
- avoid stress or major decisions
- avoid alcohol for a few days
- avoid driving alone or undertaking tiring journeys
- tell your employer or tutor that you have had a head injury
- return to work and routine daily activities gradually, avoiding overtime
- if you have problems which worry you or persist after 2 weeks, consult a doctor

After a head injury to a child

- allow the child to rest by reducing noise and light levels
- allow a few days off school
- give paracetamol for headache
- discourage noisy play or television programmes
- encourage plenty of drinks until normal appetite returns
- inform the teacher the child has had a head injury
- if your child has symptoms which worry you or persist after 2 weeks, consult a doctor

The above advice is based on head injury instructions from the Luton and Dunstable Hospital.

Road traffic accident: assessment

History
- date and time of the accident

- details of the accident

- if in a car, whether a seat belt was worn and whether there was a head restraint; whether passenger or driver

- what are the patient's descriptions of the injuries: pain, stiffness, bruising, etc

- psychological effects: shaking, insomnia, nightmares, fear of driving, flashbacks (important for compensation)

- time off work

Examination	• appropriate to affected area
	• extent of grazing and bruising – measure these
	• movement of affected limbs or neck
Tests	• none (usually)
Action	• give treatment and advice dependent on and appropriate to the injuries
	• sketch areas of grazing and bruising, or recommend a police photograph
Caution	• often the main purpose of the patient's visit is to document the injuries for a possible future compensation claim. Record the details carefully

Bites

History	• which animal?
	• immunocompromised
	• diabetes
	• prosthetic joint
Examination	• cellulitis
	• discharge
Tests	• consider wound swab
Action	• irrigate (if fresh wound)
	• give co-amoxiclav prophylactically (unless allergic to penicillin) if:
	– human, cat or complicated dog bites
	– affecting the hand or genital area

          – moderate or severe injury, crush injury or oedema

          – bone or joint penetration possible

          – immunocompromised

          – diabetes mellitus

          – affecting a prosthetic joint

- advise elevation for infected bites on arms or legs
- consider need for vaccination against tetanus and hepatitis B
- consider post-exposure prophylaxis against rabies and HIV

Refer to doctor
- allergic to penicillin
- severe wounds
- penetrating hand wound
- wounds over or near a joint
- risk of rabies

Reference

- DTB (2004) Managing bites from humans and other mammals. *Drug Ther Bull* **42**: 67–71.

9   Management of minor illness

Evidence-based practice

It is helpful for all members of a primary care team, whether in a general practice, walk-in centre or other setting, to be consistent in the way that we manage minor illness. Where differences are apparent, you should be able to access up-to-date, high-quality research evidence to aid discussion and help you to reach agreement. Critical analysis of published research has become highly complex and very time-consuming; thankfully there are now several agencies such as the Cochrane Collaboration which analyse the evidence on your behalf, and provide easy access to this information on the Internet.

Although these reviews will explore possible flaws in the published papers, there are several factors which inherently bias the whole process of evaluating evidence. They include:

- the rigorous standards and large sample sizes that are now expected in clinical trials lead to very high costs, which make it difficult to attract funding other than from pharmaceutical companies with a high turnover

- funded research is more likely to favour the sponsor's product

- negative results are less likely to be published

- old drugs may appear inadequately researched compared to new ones

- little research is conducted in primary care

- therapies that do not employ the same disease categories as Western medicine are almost impossible to research in this way

With these reservations, we recommend the following sources:

- www.prodigy.nhs.uk (excellent, evidence-based overviews; also has good patient information leaflets)

- www.library.nhs.uk (many useful resources, including the *BNF* and the Cochrane Library)

The recommendations in this book were extensively checked against Prodigy guidance at the time of writing.

Holistic care

It will be apparent from reading the other chapters of this book that the previous optimism of Western medicine about the eradication of infectious diseases by antibiotics has not been fulfilled. The more that we research these drugs, the more evidence we find that their benefits in most cases of minor illness are marginal; yet little evidence exists to support alternative treatments. Nor is it likely to be provided because, despite the recommendations of the Medical Research Council in 1997, funding for research into minor illness and the relief of self-limiting symptoms remains limited.

The nurse's first priority must be to satisfy herself that there is no evidence of serious disease, and if so to reassure the patient accordingly. This may be all that is necessary; patients do not necessarily want advice on managing their illness, and traditional nursing advice (e.g. rest, copious fluids and regular paracetamol) is not well supported by research.

It is important to be sensitive to the patient's beliefs and expectations, or 'agenda'. They may have attended in order to legitimise their illness to an employer, or at the insistence of a relative. Social factors, such as an impending holiday or examination, will often be of far greater importance to patients than any medical issues, and will inevitably influence their assessment of the relative risks and benefits of any treatment.

In Western medicine the 'placebo effect' is regarded as a nuisance which interferes with the evaluation of the 'real' effects of a treatment in clinical trials. Yet the placebo effect is itself very real, and represents the influence of the patient's belief on the intrinsic healing ability of the body. You can harness this effect very easily, by being positive and emphasising that a good recovery is likely. The placebo effect of any treatment that you suggest will be enhanced by the fact that you have recommended it, particularly if you have established a good relationship with the patient. Try to avoid destroying this effect by being too evidence based, provided that you can be sure that the treatment will do no harm. For example, writing a prescription for simple linctus while explaining 'actually, there's no evidence that this works' is unlikely to benefit the patient. Remember that any therapy that makes the patient feel better is likely to accelerate the healing process.

References

- Ernst E (2001) Towards a scientific understanding of placebo effects. In: Peters D (ed) *Understanding the Placebo Effect in Complementary Medicine*. Churchill Livingstone, Edinburgh, pp. 17–29.
- Medical Research Council (MRC) (1997) *MRC Topic Review: primary health care*. Medical Research Council, London, pp. 44–5.

Infections

The traditional Western explanation of the infectious process portrays the human body as a sterile environment that has been invaded by a hostile organism. Our scientists' efforts have been concentrated on finding newer and better chemical weapons to defeat these enemy forces. However, the spread of antibiotic resistance is causing increasing concern. Our ability to develop new antibiotics is limited; only one of the antibiotics in our formulary (clarithromycin) has been introduced within the last 20 years.

We are beginning to see that this warlike model is fundamentally flawed. The human body is more like an ecosystem, supporting a myriad of other organisms far greater in number than the cells in our body. Some of them are essential for our survival, like the intestinal bacteria which manufacture vitamin K. Broad-spectrum antibiotics dramatically alter our internal flora, leading to side-effects such as diarrhoea and vaginal thrush.

Many of the organisms that can cause infections are normal inhabitants of the healthy human body (*commensals*). The process which causes them to become pathogenic is not well understood, but often seems to be initiated by a fall in the vigilance of the immune system rather than a change in the organism itself. The immune system has intricate links with all other systems of the body, and is susceptible to the effects of nutrition and psychosocial stress. It follows from this that the maintenance of a healthy body and mind is important, both in reducing the chances of developing an infection and in speeding recovery. It also seems logical that medicines that interfere with the natural defences of the body (e.g. antipyretics, antiemetics and antidiarrhoeal drugs) should be used with caution.

Table 9.1 shows some of the bacteria that cause common infections and the antibiotics most frequently used against them.

Reference

- Guarner F and Malgelada J-R (2003) Gut flora in health and disease. *Lancet* **361**: 512–19.

Table 9.1 Some of the bacteria that cause common infections, and the antibiotics most frequently used against them

Organism	Commensal of:	Diseases	Antibiotic susceptibility
Streptococcus	Throat	Pharyngitis, otitis media, pneumonia, meningitis, cellulitis, impetigo	Penicillin V, amoxicillin, clarithromycin
Staphylococcus	Nose	Impetigo, boils, abscesses	Flucloxacillin, erythromycin, clarithromycin
Haemophilus influenzae	Upper respiratory tract	Otitis media, epiglottitis, meningitis, chest infections	Amoxicillin (80%), co-amoxiclav, erythromycin, clarithromycin, doxycycline
Escherichia coli	Intestine	UTI, abscesses, gastroenteritis	Trimethoprim, nitrofurantoin, cefalexin

Box 9.1   Recurrent infections

Sometimes patients present with a history of several different types of infection over a short period of time.

In such cases, consider:

- psychosocial stress (a potent immunosuppressant)
- increased exposure to infections (e.g. child starting school)
- white cell dysfunction (e.g. leukaemia – FBC)
- diabetes (urinalysis or fasting blood glucose)
- HIV (test with full counselling beforehand)

Reference
- Kiercolt-Glaser J *et al.* (1991) Spousal caregivers of dementia victims, changes in immunity and health. *Psychosom Med* **53**: 345.

Notifiable diseases

Diseases which must be notified to the Consultant in Communicable Disease Control (CCDC) on the appropriate form include:

- food poisoning

- suspected food poisoning

- measles

- mumps

- rubella

- pertussis

A full list is given on the cover of the book of notification forms. This notification is statutory and does not require the patient's consent. (*See* www.hpa.org.uk/confidentiality/default.htm)

Warn the patient that he or she may be contacted by the local Health Protection Unit, and explain that their role is to identify the source of infections and prevent their spread.

If there are any implications for the community, e.g. suspected food poisoning in a chef, or a rare infectious disease, notify the local consultant in communicable disease by telephone or fax.

Useful websites

- Information on infectiousness: www.hpa.org.uk/infections/topics_az/schools/schools.pdf

- *Information on rashes in pregnancy*: www.hpa.org.uk/infections/topics_az/rubella/rash.pdf

- *Information on immunoglobulin administration*: www.hpa.org.uk/infections/topics_az/immunoglobulin/pdfs/ig_handbook120704.pdf

Table 9.2 lists infectiousness and exclusion periods for common diseases, derived from information on www.hpa.org.uk.

Table 9.2 Infectiousness and exclusion periods for common diseases

Disease	Incubation period	Infective period	Exclude from school – case	Action for contacts
Chickenpox (less likely to be infectious if lesions covered)	11–20 days (chickenpox)	From 1 day before until 5 days from onset of rash	5 days after rash appears	Refer babies under 4 weeks, non-immune immunocompromised or pregnant contacts
Conjunctivitis	3–29 days	While discharge present	None	None
Diarrhoea and vomiting	1 hour–14 days (depending on cause)	While diarrhoea lasts	Until 24 h after last diarrhoea or vomiting (48 h for under 5s)	No exclusion unless bacterial cause, when CCDC will decide
Glandular fever	33–49 days	While symptomatic	Until well	None
Hand, foot and mouth disease	3–5 days	Up to 7 days	1 week or until ulcers are healed	None
Head lice	7–10 days	As long as lice or live eggs are present	Until child and family have been treated	None
Impetigo	Unknown	While purulent lesions persist	Until lesions crusted, or 48 h after treatment begun	None
Measles	6–19 days	From 4 days before onset of rash to 4 days after	5 days	Refer non-immune immunocompromised or pregnant contacts
Mumps	15–24 days	From 6 days before symptoms to 4 days after onset	5 days	None

continued overleaf

Table 9.2   Continued

Disease	Incubation period	Infective period	Exclude from school – case	Action for contacts
Parvovirus (slapped cheek)	13–18 days	Until rash appears	None	Refer pregnant contacts under 30 weeks
Pertussis (whooping cough)	5–21 days	Up to 3 weeks if untreated	5 days after starting antibiotic	None
Rubella	13–21 days	From 13 days before rash until 6 days after	5 days	Refer non-immune pregnant contacts under 20 weeks
Scabies	7–27 days	Until mites and eggs have been destroyed	Until day after treatment	None once treated
Shingles	None	Until five days after onset of rash	None, provided lesions covered	Refer babies under 4 weeks, non-immune immunocompromised or pregnant contacts if exposed to uncovered lesions
Streptococcal throat infection	12 h to 5 days	Up to 48 h after antibiotic	None, unless rash present (exclude for 5 days)	None
Threadworms	2–6 weeks	As long as eggs present on perianal skin	None once treated	None once treated
Tinea	1–2 weeks	While lesions are active	Only if epidemic suspected	None
Verrucae (plantar warts)	1–24 months	As long as wart present	None (cover wart with waterproof dressing for swimming/barefoot sports)	None

Source: Health Protection Agency, Dec 2004.

Certificates

NHS certificates

These are not issued for periods of less than 7 days: in these cases the patient should obtain an SC2 form from his or her employer, or an SC1 from the surgery if self-employed or unemployed.

The usual white certificate (MED3) is issued at the time that the patient sees a doctor. Certificates can be backdated if the patient has previously been seen by a GP, deputising service doctor or hospital doctor (pink form: MED 5). These should not be used for periods longer than one month.

No certificate can be forward-dated, although overlapping is permitted.

Closed certificates (with a return-to-work date) can only be given if the date is within 14 days of the date of issue.

Reference

• www.dwp.gov.uk/medical/faq.asp (accessed 10 June 2005).

Private certificates

These can be issued at the recommended British Medical Association (BMA) rate, which should be reclaimed from the employer.

10 Suggested specialist nurses' formulary

Notes on prescribing

Most of the drugs listed here are 'basic' and may well be included in your local formularies, policies or PGDs (Patient Group Directions), but it may be wise to cross-check. Many of these drugs can be prescribed by nurses with an extended nurse prescribing qualification, but this formulary aims to cover the range of medication commonly required to treat minor illness and is not a mirror of the extended nurse prescribers' formulary.

Drugs marked 'OTC' are available over the counter, and often cost less than a prescription charge. The price depends on the pack size, brand and pharmacy.

Prescriptions must be signed by a qualified prescriber; but if the nurse who has no such qualification can complete the details of the prescription and slip it under the prescriber's door for signature, the interruption will be minimal. Entries marked NPEF or OTC are in the Nurse Prescribers' Extended Formulary, although the indications for use under this formulary may be more limited than those covered by *The Minor Illness Manual*.

The FP10 prescription form in England has a box at the top where the number of days' treatment may be entered. This avoids the need to calculate quantities but is awkward to use. It cannot be used for variable dose drugs, creams, lotions, etc. Remember that the box is an instruction to the pharmacist as to how much to dispense, not a direction to the patient, so it will not appear on the dispensed medication instructions unless repeated in the main body of the prescription. On the whole, it is usually simpler and clearer to specify an amount to be dispensed and leave the top box blank.

The following formulary gives brief notes on the clinical use of medications and justification for recommending such medication. The *BNF* and its appendices, or the drug data sheet (formally known as the Supplementary Protection Certificate or SPC), provide more information. As a final check before giving a prescription, the acronym *PASS* can be used to check if the patient is *Pregnant, Allergic*, on *Something else*, or has a *System failure*. When considering if a patient is pregnant, bear in mind that those hoping to become pregnant but who have not yet missed a period, and mothers who are breastfeeding also need special caution when prescribing. Always check for interaction with any other current medication.

Some drugs are contraindicated, or should be given at lower dosage, to patients with kidney, liver or heart failure. If in doubt, consult a doctor.

Above all, make sure the prescription specifies the drug you intended. Most prescriptions in primary care are now computer printed. The difference between drugs with similarly spelt names can be as little as the gap between two adjacent keys on a keyboard. One of the most dangerous examples is prescribing penicillamine when penicillin was intended. Such an inadvertent swap from an antibiotic to an immunosuppressant could be fatal.

Previous antibiotic treatment

If a patient presents with a condition requiring antibiotic treatment, but has finished a course of the 'first-choice' antibiotic within the last 7 days, then either the infection is viral or the organism is resistant to the antibiotic. In these circumstances a different antibiotic may be necessary, as follows:

- for otitis media or sinusitis – change to co-amoxiclav

- for chest infections – add erythromycin or change to doxycycline (*see* notes on mycoplasma infection, page 23)

- for uncomplicated UTIs in non-pregnant women – change to either nitrofurantoin m/r or trimethoprim, whichever one was not used last time (unless sensitivities are available from the laboratory)

- for throat infections – take throat swab and await result before prescribing a different antibiotic, as in most cases the infection will be viral

Antibiotics and oral contraceptives

Broad-spectrum antibiotics (amoxicillin, co-amoxiclav, cefalexin and doxycycline) may slightly reduce the effectiveness of the COC and contraceptive patch. Advise patients to use a condom or refrain from intercourse while taking the antibiotic and for 1 week afterwards, and if there are fewer than seven pills in their packet advise them not to have a pill-free week.

Narrow-spectrum antibiotics such as penicillin V, flucloxacillin and trimethoprim do not have this effect, nor do nitrofurantoin, erythromycin or clarithromycin.

The progestogen-only pill, injection and implant are not affected by any of the antibiotics in this formulary.

Half-life (t$_{1/2}$)

The speed at which a drug is eliminated from the body is often proportional to the concentration of drug in the blood. When the drug is present in high concentration shortly after a dose, the elimination is more rapid than when it is present only in low concentration some time later. Drugs that follow this rule are said to have first-order kinetics, and they have a constant half-life. When this is so, the plasma half-life is given in this formulary. This is the time taken for the plasma concentration of the drug to reduce by one half of its starting level. It is useful to know the $t_{1/2}$ even if it is only an approximation, to help understand how long the action of a drug will last and when a further dose may be needed. When there is a known range of $t_{1/2}$ for different individuals, this is given in brackets after the mean.

Allergies

Many reported allergies are really just coincidences, for example, the appearance of a viral rash just after starting a course of antibiotic. However, any report of swelling of the tongue or face, or difficulty in breathing, must be taken seriously.

If the patient has a true allergy to one type of penicillin, *all* drugs of this class should be avoided. This does not apply if the patient experiences non-allergic side-effects, such as diarrhoea with co-amoxiclav; penicillin V will probably not produce this side-effect.

Ten percent of those allergic to penicillin will also be allergic to cephalosporins such as cefalexin.

▼ Black triangle symbol

This symbol means that there is limited experience of the use of this product and the Committee on Safety of Medicine (CSM) requests that all suspected adverse reactions should be reported. Use the yellow forms in the *BNF*. They can now be signed and submitted by any health professional, not just doctors.

◢ Less suitable for prescribing symbol

This symbol means that the Joint Formulary Committee of the *BNF* considers a drug to be 'less suitable for prescribing'. Several are in fairly common use in managing minor illnesses despite this. If you feel tempted to use a drug not in our formulary, it is worth checking to see if the *BNF* lists the drug with this symbol. If it does, then usually either there is an unacceptable balance between efficacy and side-effects, or the drug is ineffective.

Pack size

The number of tablets, capsules or items, or the volume of liquids is given in the formulary for the usual original pack dispensed. This is not to be taken as a recommendation of how much to prescribe, which depends on the patient's needs, but when possible it is more convenient for a manufactured pack to be dispensed whole, together with the patient information leaflet.

Formulary

Listed by *BNF* classification.

Gastrointestinal system

Magnesium trisilicate [1.1]
Gaviscon Advance® [1.1.2]
Ranitidine [1.3.1]
Loperamide [1.4.2]
Ispaghula husk [1.6.1]
Glycerol suppositories [1.6.2]
Senna [1.6.2]
Anusol® [1.7.1]
Xyloproct® [1.7.2]

Cardiovascular system

Tranexamic acid [2.11]

Respiratory system

Salbutamol CFC-free and Salamol Easi-Breathe® inhaler [3.1.1]
AeroChamber Plus® [3.1.5]
Peak flow meter [3.1.5]
Beclometasone inhaler and Beclazone Easi-Breathe® [3.2]
Fexofenadine [3.4.1]
Loratadine [3.4.1]
Chlorphenamine [3.4.1]
Menthol and eucalyptus [3.8]
Pholcodine [3.9.1]
Simple linctus [3.9.2]

Nervous system

Temazepam [4.1.1]
Prochlorperazine [4.6]
Domperidone [4.6]
Aspirin [4.7.1]
Paracetamol [4.7.1]
Paradote® [4.7.1]
Codeine phosphate [4.7.2]

Infections

Phenoxymethylpenicillin [5.1.1]
Flucloxacillin [5.1.1.2]
Amoxicillin [5.1.1.3]
Co-amoxiclav [5.1.1.3]
Cefalexin [5.1.2]
Doxycycline [5.1.3]
Erythromycin [5.1.5]
Clarithromycin [5.1.5]
Trimethoprim [5.1.8]
Metronidazole [5.1.11]
Nitrofurantoin m/r [5.1.13]
Fluconazole [5.2]
Nystatin [5.2]
Mebendazole [5.5.1]
Piperazine [5.5.1]

Endocrine system

Norethisterone [6.4.1.2]

Obstetrics and gynaecology

Clotrimazole [7.2.2]
Levonorgestrel [7.3.1]

Nutrition and blood

Ferrous sulphate [9.1.1]
Dioralyte® [9.2.1.2]

Musculoskeletal system

Ibuprofen [10.1.1]
Ibuprofen (topical) [10.3.2]
Algesal® [10.3.2]

Eye

Chloramphenicol [11.3.1]
Sodium cromoglicate [11.4.2]
Hypromellose [11.8.1]

Ear, nose and oropharynx

EarCalm® [12.1.1]
Otosporin® [12.1.1]
Otomize® [12.1.1]
Beclometasone aqueous spray [12.2.1]
Saline nose drops [12.2.2]
Warm moist air inhalation [12.2.2]
Chlorhexidine oral spray [12.3.4]

Skin

Emulsifying ointment [13.2.1]
Hydrous ointment [13.2.1]
Oilatum® [13.2.1.1]
Hydrocortisone [13.4]
Clobetasone butyrate [13.4]
Betamethasone valerate [13.4]

Clotrimazole/hydrocortisone [13.4]
Salicylic acid [13.7]
Sodium fusidate [13.10.1]
Clotrimazole [13.10.2]
Terbinafine [13.10.2]
Aciclovir [13.10.3]
Malathion [13.10.4]
Permethrin [13.10.4]

Gastrointestinal system

[1.1] Magnesium trisilicate (OTC)

Class:	antacid
Liquid:	magnesium trisilicate, light magnesium carbonate, sodium bicarbonate, peppermint flavour
Dose:	10 ml suspension three times daily in water
Pack:	500 ml
$t_{1/2}$:	not applicable
Side-effects:	may cause diarrhoea occasionally
Interactions:	may reduce the absorption of other drugs, for example, iron, nitrofurantoin, ciprofloxacin, fexofenadine, digoxin, phenytoin
Cautions:	as the mixture contains sodium (equivalent to about 3 level teaspoonfuls of salt in a 500 ml bottle), it should be used with caution when there is heart failure, hypertension, renal or hepatic failure
Selection:	antacids provide rapid, short-term relief from dyspepsia. Plain alkali can cause rebound acid secretion, but magnesium trisilicate forms a barrier to protect the gastric mucosa. Liquid preparations are more effective than tablets

[1.1.2] Gaviscon Advance® (OTC)

Class:	compound alginate antacid
Liquid:	sodium alginate 500 mg, potassium bicarbonate 100 mg per 5 ml
Dose:	adults and children over 12 years: 5–10 ml after meals and at bedtime
Pack:	500 ml
$t_{1/2}$:	not applicable
Side-effects:	very rarely patients sensitive to the ingredients may develop allergic manifestations such as urticaria or bronchospasm
Interactions:	as the raft is formed by the alginate and bicarbonate reacting with gastric acid to produce a froth of carbon dioxide bubbles, other medication that reduces gastric acid secretion may make a less effective raft
Cautions:	the salts of sodium, potassium and calcium (an excipient in Gaviscon Advance) might exacerbate some severe diseases, such as cardiac failure, hyperkalaemia, calcium-containing renal stones
Selection:	whereas magnesium trisilicate primarily reduces acidity and forms a barrier to protect the gastric mucosa, compound alginate agents such as Gaviscon form a raft to reduce the chance that acid can reflux up into the oesophagus, which helps to control the symptoms of mild to moderate heartburn. The Advance version has a lower sodium content than plain Gaviscon, and is no more expensive. It can be used in pregnancy

References

- Lindow SW, Regnèll P, Sykes J and Little S (2003) An open-label, multicentre study to assess the safety and efficacy of a novel reflux suppressant Gaviscon Advance in the treatment of heartburn during pregnancy. *Int J Clin Pract* **57**: 175–9.
- Chatfield S (1999) A comparison of the efficacy of the alginate preparation, Gaviscon Advance, with placebo in the treatment of gastro-oesophageal reflux disease. *Curr Med Res Opin* **15**: 152–9.

[1.3.1] Ranitidine (lower dose tablets available OTC, NPEF)

Class:	histamine (H_2) receptor antagonist
Tablets:	150 mg
Dose:	adults: 150 mg twice daily or 300 mg at night
Pack:	60
$t_{1/2}$:	2 h
Side-effects:	ranitidine is usually well tolerated, but very rarely is associated with changes in liver or kidney function, pancreatitis, reduction in white cell or platelet counts, bradycardia, headache, allergic phenomena such as rash, joint aches or vasculitis
Interactions:	none
Cautions:	the possibility of malignancy should be excluded before starting treatment with acid suppressants because they may mask symptoms of a gastric carcinoma. Use half the normal dose in severe renal impairment. Do not prescribe for people with a history of acute porphyria
Selection:	H_2 receptor antagonists provide longer-term relief from dyspeptic symptoms than antacids, and are useful for those who have already tried OTC antacids. Ranitidine rarely causes side-effects.

Reference

• Netzer P, Brabetz-Hofliger A, Brundler R et al. (1998) Comparison of the effect of the antacid Rennie versus low-dose H_2-receptor antagonists (ranitidine, famotidine) on intragastric acidity. *Aliment Pharmacol Ther* **12**: 337–42.

[1.4.2] Loperamide (OTC)

Class:	antimotility opioid
Capsules:	2 mg
Dose:	adults: two capsules initially, followed by one after each loose stool for up to a maximum of 5 days; usual dose 3–4 capsules a day, maximum of 8 capsules a day
Pack:	30
$t_{1/2}$:	11 (9–14) h
Side-effects:	abdominal cramps, bloating, nausea, vomiting and rarely paralytic ileus, dizziness, drowsiness, skin reactions
Interactions:	oral desmopressin
Cautions:	not suitable for children (although licensed from age 4), or anyone with undiagnosed abdominal pain
Selection:	loperamide provides rapid relief from diarrhoea – within 4 h for 40% of people with traveller's diarrhoea. There is a low risk of opioid abuse

References

- Wingate D, Phillips SF, Lewis SJ, Malagelada JR, Speelman P, Steffen R and Tytgat GN (2001) Guidelines for adults on self-medication for the treatment of acute diarrhoea. *Aliment Pharmacol Ther* **15**: 773–82.
- Steffen R, Heusser R, Tschopp A and Du Pont HL (1988) Efficacy and side-effects of six agents in the self-treatment of traveller's diarrhoea. *Travel Med Int* **6**: 153–7.

[1.6.1] Ispaghula husk (OTC)

Class:	bulk-forming laxative
Granules:	effervescent or non-effervescent, sugar- and gluten-free ispaghula husk, 3.5 g/sachet (plain, lemon or orange flavours available in effervescent form)
Powder:	sugar- and gluten-free ispaghula husk, 3.4 g/sachet (orange or lemon/lime flavour)
Dose:	adults: 1 sachet or 10 ml in water twice daily preferably after or with meals children 6–12 years: $1/2$ to 1 sachet or 5 ml twice daily preferably after or with meals
Pack:	30 sachets, 150 g (orange-flavoured effervescent granules), 200 g (non-effervescent plain granules)
$t_{1/2}$:	not applicable
Side-effects:	flatulence, abdominal distension, gastrointestinal obstruction or impaction, very rarely allergic reactions
Interactions:	none
Cautions:	adequate liquid intake is essential to reduce the risk of intestinal obstruction. *In vitro*, the husk can absorb up to 40 times its own weight of water. Do not prescribe for patients with difficulty swallowing, intestinal obstruction or atony, or faecal impaction
Selection:	the best form of medicine for constipation is to increase the natural fibre in the diet. When this is not achievable, bulk-forming laxatives are an alternative. Ispaghula husk is also useful for controlling diarrhoea in diverticular disease and when there is too much fluid in an ileostomy or colostomy. At first, this seems paradoxical, but it is just making use of the liquid-absorbing property of the husk

[1.6.2] Glycerol suppositories (OTC)

Class:	mildly irritant laxative
Suppositories:	gelatine 140 mg/g, glycerol 700 mg/g, purified water 160 mg/g
Dose:	adults 4 g, children 2 g, infants 1 g; insert one suppository, blunt end first, into the rectum when required
Pack:	12
$t_{1/2}$:	not applicable
Side-effects:	rectal discomfort
Interactions:	none
Selection:	glycerol is a simple, safe laxative suitable for short-term relief of distal constipation

Reference

- Abd-el-Maeboud KH, el-Naggar T, el-Hawi EM *et al.* (1991) Rectal suppository: commonsense and mode of insertion. *Lancet* **338**: 798–800.

[1.6.2] Senna (OTC)

Class:	stimulant laxative
Tablets:	7.5 mg
Liquid:	7.5 mg/5 ml
Dose:	start with the lowest dose in the range, then increase if necessary: adults: 15–30 mg at night children 6–12 years: 7.5–15 mg in the morning 2–6 years: 3.75–7.5 mg in the morning
Pack:	20 tablets, or 100 ml
$t_{1/2}$:	not applicable
Side-effects:	abdominal cramp
Interactions:	none
Cautions:	do not prescribe to patients with intestinal obstruction. Prolonged use can cause an atonic, non-functioning colon and hypokalaemia. Long-term use has this risk, but is sometimes justified. Young children with chronic constipation should be referred to a doctor
Selection:	stimulant laxative may be necessary to relieve generalised constipation where diet or a bulk-forming laxative has failed and glycerol would not help evacuate the colon. The action of senna takes about 8–12 h

[1.7.1] Anusol® (OTC)

Class:	soothing haemorrhoidal preparation
Ointment:	bismuth subgallate 2.25%, bismuth oxide 0.88%, balsam peru 1.88%, zinc oxide 10.75%
Suppositories:	similar proportions as above in a 2.8 g suppository
Dose:	one suppository or application of ointment night and morning and after defaecation
Pack:	12 or 24 suppositories, 1 × 25 g of ointment
$t_{1/2}$:	not applicable
Side-effects:	rarely discomfort on application or local dermatitis
Interactions:	none
Cautions:	avoid prescribing to patients who are sensitive to lanolin as this is one of the excipients
Selection:	Anusol exerts its effects locally without systemic absorption. Although no formal trial in pregnancy has been done, it has been used during pregnancy for many years and is considered safe. The ointment is used for external haemorrhoids and may provide better protection and lubrication of the anal surface than a cream. Suppositories are used for internal haemorrhoids

[1.7.2] Xyloproct®

Class:	soothing haemorrhoidal preparation with cortico-steroid and local anaesthetic
Ointment:	aluminium acetate 3.5%, hydrocortisone acetate 0.275%, lidocaine 5%, zinc oxide 18%
Dose:	apply several times daily
Pack:	20 g
$t_{1/2}$:	not applicable
Side-effects:	stinging on application, local dermatitis, very rarely systemic effects from absorption of the components, with confusion in children or hypersensitivity reactions
Cautions:	pregnancy, anal infections such as *Herpes simplex* or candida. Avoid prolonged use which could theoretically result in local skin atrophy from the hydrocortisone. It would be very unusual to pre-scribe this for a child
Selection:	the idea is that the corticosteroid controls itching and the lidocaine controls the pain. The aluminium acetate is a soothing component. An applicator is supplied so that the ointment can be applied within the rectum if required. The usual indication is painful or irritant haemorrhoids, but the preparation is also useful for symptomatic relief from an anal fissure or troublesome pruritus ani

Cardiovascular system

[2.11] Tranexamic acid

Class:	Antifibrinolytic (inhibits the natural destruction of fibrin in clots)
Tablets:	500 mg
Dose:	adults: 2 tablets three times a day
Pack:	60
$t_{1/2}$:	2 h after intravenous (IV) injection (the duration of action of tablets will depend on the rate of absorption)
Side-effects:	nausea, vomiting, diarrhoea (these often resolve if the dose is reduced), disturbance of colour vision (discontinue), rarely thrombotic events (discontinue)
Interactions:	counteracts fibrinolytic drugs, such as streptokinase
Cautions:	do not prescribe to anyone with a history of thromboembolic disease. Lower doses are required in renal impairment. There is no evidence of harm during pregnancy or breast-feeding, but the manufacturer advises caution
Selection:	this is one of the few non-hormonal treatments for menorrhagia. Tranexamic acid causes a greater reduction of heavy menstrual bleeding and no increase in side-effects when compared with placebo or other medical therapies (NSAIDS, oral progestogens and etamsylate). It is probably underused because of misplaced fears about causing thrombosis. Long-term studies in Sweden have shown that the rate of thrombosis in women treated with tranexamic acid is comparable with the spontaneous backgound frequency

Reference

- Lethaby A, Farquhar C and Cooke I (2000) Antifibrinolytics for heavy menstrual bleeding (Cochrane Review). *The Cochrane Library, Issue 4, 2000.* Update Software, Oxford.

Respiratory system

[3.1.1] Salbutamol CFC-free and Salamol Easi-Breathe® inhaler (NPEF)

Class:	β₂ adrenoceptor agonist (mimics the action of adrenaline at the β₂ receptors in the lungs)
Inhaler:	100 μg per dose
Nebuliser solution:	2.5 mg/2.5 ml, 5 mg/2.5 ml
Dose:	inhaler: adult 2 doses, child 1–2 doses nebuliser: adult 5 mg, child 2.5 mg These doses can be repeated up to four times in a day if required, but follow the BTS asthma guidelines for appropriate treatment of persistent symptoms
Pack:	1 inhaler or 20 ampoules of nebuliser solution
$t_{1/2}$:	5 (4–6) h
Side-effects:	fine tremor (particularly hands), nervous tension, headache, tachycardia, hypokalaemia, disturbance of sleep and behaviour in children, allergic reactions including paradoxical broncho-spasm with exacerbation of wheezing shortly after receiving a dose of salbutamol (discontinue and substitute ipratropium bromide)
Interactions:	high doses of salbutamol can cause dangerous hypokalaemia, particularly in combination with corticosteroids, diuretics, theophylline or hypoxia. Patients needing salbutamol should not be taking a beta-blocker (which has the opposite action), especially a non-selective one such as propranolol. Salbutamol possibly reduces plasma concentration of digoxin
Cautions:	patients finding that salbutamol is not relieving their symptoms should seek medical advice and be treated according to the BTS guidelines. Increasing frequency of use of salbutamol suggests

continued opposite

deteriorating asthma in need of anti-inflammatory treatment with inhaled or oral corticosteroids. Caution is needed when prescribing for patients with hyperthyroidism, ischaemic heart disease, arrhythmias, hypertension, or any predisposing factors to hypokalaemia

Selection:

Short-acting β_2 adrenoceptor agonists are the first step in the management of asthma. Nebulisers offer no advantage over spacer devices for delivery, but some patients, who are either young children or frightened adults, find the nebuliser easier. Ideally use a spacer device. If you have to use a nebuliser, it should be driven by pressurised oxygen. Easi-Breathe is the inhaler device most liked by patients, but is several times the cost of the standard inhaler when it contains salbutamol, however the steroid versions are the same price. If the patient uses a regular inhaled steroid, prescribe the same type of inhaler for their salbutamol

References

- Cates CJ, Bara A, Crilly JA and Rowe BH (2003) Holding chambers versus nebulisers for beta-agonist treatment of acute asthma (Cochrane Review). *The Cochrane Library, Issue 2, 2003*. Update Software, Oxford.
- Lenney J, Innes JA and Crompton GK (2000) Inappropriate inhaler use: assessment of use and patient preference of seven inhalation devices. *Resp Med* **94**: 496–500.

[3.1.5] AeroChamber Plus® (OTC)

Class:	medium-sized spacer device
Device:	standard adult (blue), with mask (blue), child device with mask (yellow), infant device with mask (orange)
Cautions:	advise that the device should be washed no more often than once a month and is best left to dry in the air because wiping with a cloth creates a static electric charge on the plastic which can affect drug delivery. Replace the device every year
Selection:	spacer devices reduce the need for co-ordination when using metered dose inhalers and slow the speed of the aerosol spray, improving the deposition of the drug in the lungs, with less being sprayed directly onto the back of the throat. However, a study in the elderly concluded that breath-activated and dry powder inhalers were more likely to be used correctly than metered-dose inhalers with large volume spacers. AeroChamber Plus works with a wide variety of inhalers and is available in a range to suit children. The *BNF* says that larger devices with one-way valves work better, but a systematic review of inhaler devices shows no difference in efficacy. In our experience, any theoretical advantage of large volume spacers may be outweighed by problems with compliance. The noise of the valve moving in the large spacers disturbs some younger users, and adults find them cumbersome to use anywhere away from home

References

- Jones V, Fernandez C and Diggory P (1999) A comparison of large volume spacer, breath-activated and dry powder inhalers in older people. *Age Ageing* **28**: 481–4.
- MeReC (1995) Inhaler devices: an update. *MeReC Bulletin* **6**: 1–4.
- Centre for Reviews and Dissemination. Inhaler devices for the management of asthma and COPD. Centre for Reviews and Dissemination, York, **12**.

[3.1.5] Peak flow meter (OTC)

Class: disease-monitoring device

Device: standard range for adults and children, low range for adults who can only manage peak flows less than 400 l/minute or children

Cautions: children under 5 years of age cannot reliably use a peak flow meter, and older ones cannot be expected to keep an accurate record of their readings

Selection: all peak flow meters available on an NHS prescription now conform to a European standard (EN 13826), so it does not matter which one you choose. (Part of the standard is that the meter should measure flows up to 800 l/min, technically all paediatric meters fail to conform, but the point is academic.) Standard ranges of peak flow have changed to match the new meters. Details can be found at www.peakflow.com. A small digital device (Piko-1) is now available at a slightly higher cost. An asthma management plan, whereby the patient knows what to do if their condition starts to deteriorate, is what matters, rather than whether it is based on symptoms or peak flow readings

References

- Powell H and Gibson PG (2002) Options for self-management education for adults with asthma (Cochrane Review). *The Cochrane Library, Issue 3, 2002.* Update Software, Oxford.
- Kamps AW, Roorda RJ and Brand PL (2001) Peak flow diaries in childhood asthma are unreliable. *Thorax* **56**: 180–2.

[3.2] Beclometasone inhaler and Beclazone Easi-Breathe®

Class:	inhaled adrenocortical steroid
Inhaler:	50, 100 and (in the standard inhaler only) 200 μg per dose
Dose:	*see* text on acute asthma (page 24), 100–800 μg/day
Pack:	200-dose inhaler
$t_{1/2}$:	30 minutes. What matters clinically is that the time to maximum effect of the first dose is 2–8 h by whatever route the adrenocortical steroid is administered. Maximum effect of repeated doses of inhaled beclometasone may not be achieved for 3 to 7 days
Side-effects:	may precipitate oral thrush (in which case use a spacer and rinse mouth after use); rarely: paradoxical bronchospasm, glaucoma, cataracts
Interactions:	none
Cautions:	tuberculosis (quiescent disease may be reactivated), high doses may induce adrenal suppression (patients on doses over 800 μg/day should be issued with a steroid card), children's height monitored and adults considered for monitoring of bone mineral density
Selection:	at equipotent doses, the type of adrenocortical steroid makes no difference to its effectiveness. This is the reason why national guidelines recommend prescribing the cheapest. The delivery system should suit the patient and there is virtually no difference in cost between the standard and the Easi-Breathe steroid inhalers

Reference

• Iwasaki E and Baba M (1993) [Pharmacokinetics and pharmacodynamics of hydrocortisone in asthmatic children]. [Japanese] *Arerugi – Japanese Journal of Allergology* **42**: 1555–62.

[3.4.1] Fexofenadine (NPEF)

Class:	histamine (H_1) receptor blocker
Tablets:	120 mg
Dose:	adults and children over 12 years: 120 mg once a day children 6–11 years: 30 mg twice a day
Pack:	30 (120 mg tablets); 60 (30 mg tablets)
$t_{1/2}$:	14 (11–15) h
Side-effects:	incidence of sedation is low but it is still worth warning drivers to be alert to the slight possibility of drowsiness or dizziness
Interactions:	erythromycin and ketoconazole increase plasma levels of fexofenadine by 2 to 3 times, but no adverse effects of this are reported. Antacids containing aluminium or magnesium hydroxide (not trisilicate) are known to reduce absorption of fexofenadine (use an alternative antacid or leave 2 h between the antacid and the fexofenadine doses). Theoretical antagonism of betahistine
Cautions:	pregnancy, breast-feeding, porphyria
Selection:	fexofenadine is the active metabolite of terfenadine, but free of its potential to induce arrhythmias. So if the patient says that terfenadine used to control their hay fever well, try fexofenadine. All non-sedating antihistamines have a low risk of causing drowsiness, but fexofenadine and loratadine have a lower incidence of sedation than cetirizine or acrivastine

Reference

- Mann RD, Pearce GL, Dunn N, Shakir S and Ferner RE (2000) Sedation with 'non-sedating' antihistamines: four prescription-event monitoring studies in general practice. *BMJ* **320**: 1184–7.

[3.4.1] Loratadine (OTC)

Class:	histamine (H_1) receptor blocker
Tablets:	10 mg
Liquid:	5 mg/5 ml
Dose:	adults and children over 6 years: 10 mg daily children 2–5 years: 5 mg daily
Pack:	30 tablets; 100 ml liquid
$t_{1/2}$:	15 h
Side-effects:	incidence of sedation is low but it is still worth warning drivers to be alert to the slight possibility of drowsiness or dizziness
Interactions:	cimetidine, erythromycin, ketoconazole and possibly fluconazole, fluoxetine, amprenavir and quinidine, may increase plasma levels of loratadine or the interacting drug, and could cause adverse effects from either. Theoretical antagonism of betahistine
Cautions:	pregnancy, breast-feeding

[3.4.1] Chlorphenamine (OTC)

Class:	histamine (H$_1$) receptor blocker
Tablets:	4 mg
Liquid:	2 mg/5 ml
Dose:	although the doses below are quoted in the *BNF*, the long half-life of chlorphenamine means that a single dose can suffice in most individuals adults: 4 mg every 4–6 h, maximum 24 mg daily children 1–2 years: 1 mg twice a day 2–5 years: 1 mg every 4–6 h, maximum 6 mg daily 6–12 years: 2 mg every 4–6 h, maximum 12 mg daily
Pack:	any number of tablets (usually about 20); 150 ml liquid
$t_{1/2}$:	18 (11–33) h, with considerable variability between individuals
Side-effects:	drowsiness may affect performance of skilled tasks, e.g. driving; headache, psychomotor impairment, dry mouth, blurred vision, urinary retention and gastrointestinal disturbances; occasionally allergic reactions such as rashes or photosensitivity; rarely paradoxical stimulation. Children and elderly people are particularly susceptible to side-effects
Interactions:	sedatives (including alcohol), monoamine oxidase inhibitors (MAOIs) and tricyclic antidepressants, quinidine
Cautions:	prostatic hypertrophy, urinary retention, glaucoma, hepatic or renal disease, epilepsy. Allow enough time for the effects to wear off before the patient returns to any activity that could be dangerous under sedation

continued overleaf

Selection: chlorphenamine is useful when sedation is helpful, such as disruption of sleep caused by skin irritation or cough. The sedative effect is not mediated by blocking histamine, but by other actions of the drug

References

- Yasuda SU, Zannikos P, Young AE *et al.* (2002) The roles of CYP2D6 and stereoselectivity in the clinical pharmacokinetics of chlorpheniramine. *Br J Clin Pharmacol* **53**(5): 519–25.
- Simons KJ, Martin TJ, Watson WT and Simons FE (1990) Pharmacokinetics and pharmacodynamics of terfenadine and chlorpheniramine in the elderly. *J Allergy Clin Immunol* **85**: 540–7.

[3.8] Menthol and eucalyptus (OTC)

Class: aromatic inhalation

Liquid: race- or levo- menthol 2 g, eucalyptus oil 10 ml, light magnesium carbonate 7 g, water to 100 ml

Dose: add one teaspoonful to a pint of hot water and inhale vapour

Pack: 100 ml

Side-effects: only scalds from spilling the water

Interactions: none

Cautions: use hot, not boiling, water, may induce apnoea in infants less than 3 months

Selection: the ingredients encourage the inhalation of water vapour, which can be soothing in bronchitis or sinusitis, and may also have a useful placebo action. Inhaler devices are available for about £7 which may reduce the risk of scalding

[3.9.1] Pholcodine (OTC)

Class:	cough suppressant
Linctus:	5 mg/5 ml or 10 mg/5 ml (sugar-free available)
Dose:	adults: 5–10 mg, three to four times daily
Pack:	100 ml
$t_{1/2}$:	50 (32–54) h
Side-effects:	may dry the bronchial mucosa and thicken sputum; constipation; in large doses respiratory depression
Interactions:	sedatives (including alcohol), mexiletine, MAOIs, antidepressants
Cautions:	asthma, hepatic and renal impairment, history of drug abuse
Selection:	before prescribing, ask yourself if it is appropriate to try to reduce the coughing. Adults may be distressed by a dry, unproductive cough. Pholcodine, as the name suggests, is an opioid. Part of the antitussive effect is by sedation of the central nervous system part of the cough reflex. In children, coughing is usually helpful, but if necessary a sedative antihistamine is more effective at providing some rest at night than pholcodine. Note the long half-life means that doses could be less frequent than usually recommended

References

- Chen ZR, Bochner F and Somogyi A (1988) Pharmacokinetics of pholcodine in healthy volunteers: single and chronic dosing studies. *Br J Clin Pharmacol* **26**: 445–53.
- Findlay JW (1988) Pholcodine. [Review] *J Clin Pharma Ther* **13**: 5–17.

[3.9.2] Simple linctus (OTC)

Class:	demulcent cough linctus
Linctus:	adults: citric acid monohydrate 2.5% in a suitable vehicle with anise flavour; children: citric acid monohydrate 0.625% in a suitable vehicle with anise flavour
Dose:	adults: 5 ml of adult linctus four times daily children 6–12 years: 10 ml of paediatric linctus four times daily 2–5 years: 5 ml of paediatric linctus four times daily
Pack:	100 ml
$t_{1/2}$:	not applicable
Side-effects:	none
Interactions:	none
Cautions:	none
Selection:	a demulcent is a substance that coats mucous membranes to allay irritation. Simple linctus contains soothing substances that may help patients to tolerate a dry irritating cough without any risk of side-effects. Note this is quite different from expectorants, which aim to promote the coughing up of sputum. There is no evidence of effectiveness of any OTC cough linctus. Quite often patients attend because of a persisting cough for which they are taking an expectorant-type of cough medicine inappropriately; all that is required is to stop the expectorant

References

- Schroeder K and Fahey T (2002) Should we advise parents to administer over the counter cough medicines for acute cough? Systematic review of randomised controlled trials. *Arch Dis Child* **86**: 170–5.
- Schroeder K and Fahey T (2002) Systematic review of randomised controlled trials of over the counter cough medicines for acute cough in adults. *BMJ* **324**: 329–31.

Nervous system

[4.1.1] Temazepam

Class:	benzodiazepine hypnotic
Tablets:	10 mg
Dose:	one at night
Pack:	28, but limit prescriptions to 7 tablets
$t_{1/2}$:	men: 8 (7–15) h, women: 17 h, overall range: 7–38 h
Side-effects:	drowsiness and lightheadedness the next day; confusion, paradoxical agitation and ataxia (especially in the elderly); addiction from long-term use
Interactions:	enhanced sedation with other sedatives including alcohol, opiates, tricyclic antidepressants, antihistamines, antipsychotics, disulfiram, lofexidine, baclofen, tizanidine, cimetidine
Cautions:	potentially addictive, may cause daytime drowsiness the following day and affect driving, enhances the effect of alcohol. Do not use in those with chronic chest disease, liver or renal disease, or in pregnancy or breastfeeding
Selection:	hypnotics are occasionally very useful for short-term relief of insomnia – usually related to psychological stress, but are not suitable for long-term use because of the risk of addiction and the fact that there is often a better, non-pharmacological, solution to the problem. Temazepam has the advantage of being one of the shorter acting hypnotics and is therefore less likely to cause drowsiness the next day, although it is not free of this risk, particularly in women. Be careful to warn patients that it may impair their driving ability the next morning. Age does not seem to affect the duration of action of the drug, but the elderly are more susceptible to side-effects. Tolerance does not appear to be a problem

continued overleaf

References

- Divoll M, Greenblatt DJ, Harmatz JS and Shader RI (1981) Effect of age and gender on disposition of temazepam. *J Pharm Sci* **70**: 1104–7.
- van Steveninck AL, Wallnofer AE, Schoemaker RC *et al.* (1997) A study of the effects of long-term use on individual sensitivity to temazepam and lorazepam in a clinical population. *Br J Clin Pharmacol* **44**: 267–75.

[4.6] Prochlorperazine (buccal tablets OTC to people over 18 years, limited amount)

Class:	phenothiazide type anti-emetic
Tablets:	5 mg
Buccal tablets:	3 mg
Liquid:	5 mg/5 ml
Suppositories:	5, 25 mg
Dose:	adults only tablets/liquid labyrinthitis: 5 mg three times daily initially acute nausea/vomiting: 20 mg initially, 10 mg after 2 h prevention of nausea/vomiting: 5–10 mg three times daily buccal tablets: 1 or 2 tablets twice a day, place high between upper lip and gum and leave to dissolve (buccal 3 mg twice daily is equivalent to an oral dose of 5 mg three times daily) suppositories: 25 mg inserted into rectum followed by oral dose after 6 h as above *or* for migraine, 5 mg suppository three times a day
Pack:	no specific pack size of tablets (usually about 20); 100 ml liquid; 10 suppositories; 50 buccal tablets
$t_{1/2}$:	8 (6–10) h
Side-effects:	for a full list see the *BNF* under chlorpromazine, but in practice the only common one is drowsiness, and very occasionally severe dystonic reactions (*see* below)

continued opposite

Interactions: enhanced sedation with other sedatives including alcohol, desferrioxamine, dopaminergic drugs in Parkinson's disease (e.g. levodopa), lithium

Cautions: may cause severe dystonic reactions (abnormal face and body movements). This is rare, but more common in teenagers and young adults (acute 'oculogyric' reactions), the elderly (delayed Parkinsonian-type reactions), and the risk may be exacerbated by a concurrent viral illness. It is therefore wise to avoid prescribing prochlorperazine for these groups

Selection: prochlorperazine is useful when sedation is helpful in addition to an anti-emetic action. Often the distress of feeling nauseous is a major part of the problem and a degree of sedation is welcome. As the end of the drug name implies, this belongs to the phenothiazine group of drugs, other members of which are used as antipsychotics. Thus it is no surprise that prochlorperazine is liable to give rise to central nervous system side-effects, and this is what limits its use

References

- Isah AO, Rawlins MD and Bateman DN (1991) Clinical pharmacology of prochlorperazine in healthy young males. *Br J Clin Pharmacol* **32**: 677–84.
- Schumock GT and Martinez E (1991) Acute oculogyric crisis after administration of prochlorperazine. *South Med J* **84**: 407–8.
- Hessell PG, Lloyd-Jones JG, Muir NC, Parr GD and Sugden K (1989) A comparison of the availability of prochlorperazine following i.m., buccal and oral administration. *Int J Pharmaceutics* **52**: 159–64.

[4.6] Domperidone (OTC, limited amount, promoted for dyspepsia rather than nausea, NPEF)

Class:	dopamine (D_2) receptor blocker
Tablets:	10 mg
Liquid:	5 mg/5 ml
Suppositories:	30 mg
Dose:	adults only: oral: 10–20 mg every 4–8 h rectal: 60 mg twice daily
Pack:	30 tablets; 200 ml liquid; 10 suppositories
$t_{1/2}$:	7 h
Side-effects:	raised prolactin concentrations (possible breast tissue enlargement and leakage of milk from the nipples); occasionally reduced libido and, very rarely acute dystonic reactions
Interactions:	antagonised by opioid analgesics, increased absorption of paracetamol
Cautions:	avoid in liver disease and pregnancy, reduce dose in renal impairment
Selection:	because domperidone does not cross the blood–brain barrier, the acute dystonic reactions seen with metoclopramide and prochlorperazine are much less likely to occur. It blocks peripheral D_2 receptors, including those in the chemoreceptor trigger zone. It is a logical choice to minimise drug-induced nausea (e.g. associated with post-coital contraception) when sedation is not required and minimising the risk of side-effects is paramount

Reference

• Barone JA (1999) Domperidone: a peripherally acting dopamine2-receptor antagonist. [Review] *Ann Pharmacother* **33**: 429–40.

[4.7.1] Aspirin (OTC)

Class:	antiplatelet agent
Tablets:	75 mg, 300 mg (dispersible also available)
Dose:	adults, ideally taken with or after food anti-thrombotic use 75–300 mg daily (usually 75 mg daily for long-term use, and 300 mg as the first dose for acute chest pain)
Pack:	28
$t_{1/2}$:	2–3 h, but the effect of 300 mg lasts up to 3 days
Side-effects:	high incidence of gastrointestinal irritation with slight asymptomatic blood loss, increased bleeding time, bronchospasm and skin reactions in hypersensitive patients
Interactions:	important interaction with warfarin, avoid co-prescribing with NSAIDs or methotrexate, increased risk of bleeding with selective serotonin reuptake inhibitor (SSRI), antidepressants, clopidogrel or adrenocorticosteroids
Cautions:	*not for use by children under 16 years*; caution in those with allergy, peptic ulcer, gout, pregnancy, breastfeeding, asthma (a small proportion of asth-matic patients find that aspirin worsens their symptoms; occasionally this can be severe)
Selection:	aspirin disables an enzyme essential to the action of platelets sticking together. As platelets have no cell nucleus, they never recover this ability, but 10% of the platelet population is replaced daily. A single dose of 300 mg inhibits all platelets, 75 mg inhibits about 30% and can be used to maintain antiplatelet action. Platelet function is restored to near normal 24 h after stopping aspirin by the 10% of newly formed platelets, so missing a dose or two can cause the protection against strokes and heart attacks to be lost

Reference

- Furukawa K and Hitoshi O (2004) Inhibition of platelet aggregation with aspirin falls quickly at 1 day after discontinuation and vanished after 3 days. *J Thorac Cardiovasc Surg* **127**: 1814–15.

[4.7.1] Paracetamol (OTC)

Class:	non-opioid analgesic
Tablets:	500 mg
Soluble tablets:	500 mg Paediatric soluble tablets: 120 mg
Liquid:	250 mg/5 ml, 120 mg/5 ml
Suppositories:	60, 125, 250, 500 mg
Dose:	all up to four times a day, by mouth or by rectum adults: 500–1000 mg children 6–12 years: 250–500 mg 1–5 years: 120–250 mg 3 months–1 year: 60–120 mg
Pack:	no specific pack size of tablets (usually about 28); 100 ml liquid; 10 suppositories
$t_{1/2}$:	2 (1–3) h
Side-effects:	overdose is the only serious problem
Interactions:	prolonged regular use possibly enhances warfarin, colestyramine reduces absorption of paracetamol, whereas metoclopramide, domperidone and sodium bicarbonate can accelerate it
Cautions:	overdosage with paracetamol is particularly dangerous as it may cause hepatic damage which is sometimes not apparent for 4 to 6 days. Legislation to limit the pack sizes available over the counter has reduced the number of deaths and large overdoses, so prescribing a limited supply for acute self-limiting conditions may help achieve the same aim. Pre-existing liver disease or taking enzyme-inducing drugs (including alcohol) makes the potential for toxic effects greater. Although paracetamol is often given to babies under 3 months of age to prevent or treat post-immunisation pyrexia, it is questionable whether this is necessary. Neonates absorb and eliminate paracetamol differently from older children and adults, but toxic effects from paracetamol are most unlikely

continued opposite

Selection: paracetamol is virtually free of side-effects when
                        taken in the normal dose range

References

- Arana A, Morton NS and Hansen TG (2001) Treatment with paracetamol in infants. [Review] *Acta Anaesthesiol Scand* **45**: 20–9.
- Isbister GK, Bucens IK and Whyte IM (2001) Paracetamol overdose in a preterm neonate. *Arch Dis Child Fetal Neonatal Ed* **85**: F70–F72.
- Hawton K, Simkin S, Deeks J *et al.* (2004) UK legislation on analgesic packs: before and after study of long term effect on poisonings *BMJ* **329**: 1076–9.

[4.7.1] Paradote® (OTC)

Class: non-opioid analgesic

Tablets: 500 mg paracetamol, 100 mg methionine

Dose: adults: 500–1000 mg up to four times a day

Pack: 24

$t_{1/2}$:   2 (1–3) h (paracetamol)

Side-effects: most unlikely

Interactions: as for paracetamol, plus levodopa and MAOI-type
                        antidepressants

Cautions: liver or renal disease, pregnancy or lactation

Selection: paracetamol is involved in 20% of all deaths from
                        overdose and poisoning in England and Wales, and
                        is the only drug taken in an average of 175 cases
                        of fatal overdose per year. If you have *any* concern
                        about prescribing paracetamol to a person at risk,
                        consider discussing with them the option of
                        Paradote, which contains the antidote methionine

Reference

- Zakyeya A and Majeed A (2000) Paracetamol related deaths in England and Wales, 1993–97. *Health Statistics Quarterly, London* **7**: 5–9.

[4.7.2] Codeine phosphate

Class:	opioid analgesic
Tablets:	30 mg
Dose:	adults: 30 mg when required up to 4-hourly
Pack:	no specific pack size of tablets (usually about 20)
$t_{1/2}$:	3 h
Side-effects:	constipation, nausea, dependence, may cause drowsiness, respiratory depression, hypotension, difficulty with micturition and a variety of rare side-effects listed in the *BNF* under morphine
Interactions:	sedatives (including alcohol), MAOI-type anti-depressants, cimetidine, reduced action of domperidone and metoclopramide on the gut
Cautions:	avoid in significant respiratory, renal or liver (including biliary) disease, or after a head injury, or in the third trimester of pregnancy; may exacerbate urinary obstructive symptoms, or confusion in elderly or debilitated. To take this drug abroad, patients may require a letter from their doctor stating that it is a necessary medication
Selection:	codeine is effective at improving the analgesia provided by paracetamol, but only if it is taken in an adequate dose. The best dose to balance effectiveness against side-effects is 30 mg. Fixed combination tablets contain paracetamol/codeine in ratios of 500/8 mg or 500/30 mg, which makes it impossible to achieve the best dose of each analgesic. In prescribing codeine separately, you can give the patient the freedom to match the analgesic they take to the degree of pain: paracetamol alone for mild pain, codeine alone for more moderate, or both for more severe pain. Minimising the need to take the codeine with every dose minimises the side-effects. Dihydrocodeine offers no advantages over codeine. The codeine group of analgesics can increase biliary spasm, so are not suitable to relieve biliary colic. NSAIDs (such as ibuprofen) are preferable for inflammatory conditions, or dental pain

continued opposite

References

- Moore A, Collins S, Carroll D and McQuay H (1997) Paracetamol with and without codeine in acute pain: a quantitative systematic review. [Review] *Pain* **70**: 193–201.
- Mehlisch D, Frakes L, Cavaliere MB and Gelman M (1984) Double-blind parallel comparison of single oral doses of ketoprofen, codeine, and placebo in patients with moderate to severe dental pain. *J Clin Pharmacol* **24**: 486–92.

Infections

[5.1.1] Phenoxymethylpenicillin (Penicillin V)

Class:	narrow-spectrum, bactericidal antibiotic
Tablets:	250 mg
Liquid:	125 mg/5 ml, 250 mg/5 ml
Dose:	all four times a day, an hour before food or on an empty stomach adults: 500 mg, increased to 1000 mg in severe infections children 6–12 years: 250 mg 1–5 years: 125 mg up to 1 year: 62.5 mg
Pack:	28; 100 ml; but the usual prescription for strepto-coccal tonsillitis in adults is 80 tablets
$t_{1/2}$:	45 (30–60) minutes
Side-effects:	hypersensitivity reactions including urticaria, fever, joint pains, rashes, angio-oedema, and in severe cases anaphylaxis; interstitial nephritis; antibiotic-associated diarrhoea, reduction in platelet, white or red blood cell counts, increased risk of bleeding, rarely convulsions
Interactions:	phenoxymethylpenicillin is not a broad-spectrum antibiotic and therefore does not affect the combined oral contraceptive or warfarin
Cautions:	penicillin allergy, lower doses may be needed in renal impairment

continued overleaf

Selection:	phenoxymethylpenicillin is useful for treating strep-tococcal tonsillitis, but the absorption is too variable for the antibiotic to be reliably used for serious infections or those needing fast onset of action. Note the adult dose recommended by authorities in the UK starts at 500 mg four times daily. Otherwise the variable absorption can result in subtherapeutic blood level, leading to treatment failure and the risk of developing resistant bacteria. Prescribing a 10-day course may reduce the chance of recurrence of the infection

References

- Scottish Intercollegiate Guidelines Network (SIGN) www.sign.ac.uk/guidelines/fulltext/34/section5.html (accessed 13 June 2005).
- British Medical Association and Royal Pharmaceutical Society of Great Britain (2004) *British National Formulary*. British Medical Association and Royal Pharmaceutical Society of Great Britain, London, **48**: 270.

[5.1.1.2] Flucloxacillin (NPEF)

Class:	β-lactamase-resistant narrow-spectrum bactericidal antibacterial
Capsules:	250, 500 mg
Oral solution:	125 mg/5 ml, 250 mg/5 ml
Dose:	all four times a day, an hour before food or on an empty stomach, doses may be doubled in severe infection adults and children over 10 years: 250 mg children 2–10 years: 125 mg up to 2 years: 62.5 mg
Pack:	no specific number of capsules per pack, liquid 100 ml, but usual prescription is for 28 capsules, or 140 ml of liquid
$t_{1/2}$:	1 h
Side-effects:	see phenoxymethylpenicillin above; rarely hepatitis, cholestatic jaundice which can develop several weeks after the course (the risk is greater for courses longer than two weeks and for older patients)
Interactions:	flucloxacillin is a narrow-spectrum antibiotic and therefore does not affect the combined oral contraceptive or warfarin
Cautions:	penicillin allergy, porphyria, children may not like the taste – co-amoxiclav is then an alternative, though broader spectrum
Selection:	this is the standard treatment against staphylococcal infections

References

- Miros M, Kerlin P, Walker N and Harris O (1990) Flucloxacillin induced delayed cholestatic hepatitis. Aust N Z J Med **20**: 251–3.
- Matsui D, Barron A and Rieder MJ (1996) Assessment of the palatability of antistaphylococcal antibiotics in pediatric volunteers. Ann Pharmacother **30**: 586–8.

[5.1.1.3] Amoxicillin (NPEF)

Class:	broad-spectrum, bactericidal antibacterial
Capsules:	250, 500 mg
Liquid:	125 mg/1.25 ml, 125 mg/5 ml, 250 mg/5 ml
Dose:	for general infections: dose three times a day, may be doubled in severe infection adults and children over 10 years: 250 mg children up to 10 years: 125 mg *or* for dental abscess in adults: 3 g repeated after 8 h
Pack:	21; 100 ml; 20 ml of paediatric liquid 125 mg/1.25 ml
$t_{1/2}$:	1 h
Side-effects:	nausea, diarrhoea, rashes, allergic reactions; also *see* phenoxymethylpenicillin above
Interactions:	warfarin effect may be altered, slight reduction in efficacy of combined oral contraceptive pill
Cautions:	allergy, glandular fever (may cause rash), reduce dose in renal impairment
Selection:	amoxicillin is a broad-spectrum antibacterial suitable for treating a wide variety of infections. It is better absorbed than ampicillin and not affected by food. The paediatric liquid (125 mg/1.25 ml) is available in peach, strawberry and lemon flavours; the standard liquid is banana flavoured. The choice may help concordance but we have found no research into this, which is surprising given the 29% non-concordance reported for amoxicillin liquids taken by children. The cost of the paediatric liquid (125 mg/1.25 ml) is three times more than the standard liquid form

References

- Hoppe JE and Wahrenberger C (1999) Compliance of pediatric patients with treatment involving antibiotic suspensions: A pilot study. *Clin Ther* **21**: 1193–201.
- Adam D (1994) Advances in the treatment with amoxicillin in childhood. *Sozialpadiatrie und Kinderarztliche Praxis* **16**: 463–6.

[5.1.1.3] Co-amoxiclav

Class:	β-lactamase-resistant broad-spectrum bactericidal antibacterial; a combination of amoxicillin and clavulanic acid
Tablets:	250/125 mg (= 375 mg) or 500/125 mg (= 625 mg)
Liquid:	400/57 mg in 5 ml
Dose:	adults: 375 mg three times a day, increased to 625 mg in severe infections children using 400/57 mg suspension: (be careful to specify the strength of the suspension as there are several types) 7–12 years: 5 ml twice a day 2–6 years: 2.5 ml twice a day 2 months–2 years: 0.15 ml *per kg* twice a day
Pack:	21; 35, 70 ml
$t_{1/2}$:	1 h (amoxicillin)
Side-effects:	nausea, diarrhoea, rashes, hepatitis, cholestatic jaundice: 1 in 6000 risk of liver damage (greater risk in men over 65 years of age, and with courses lasting over 2 weeks, but rare in children); also *see* phenoxymethylpenicillin above
Interactions:	warfarin effect may be altered, slight reduction in efficacy of combined oral contraceptive pill
Cautions:	penicillin allergy, liver or renal impairment
Selection:	clavulanic acid is itself a β-lactam and can distract β-lactamase away from penicillins by acting as a suicide inhibitor, swamping the enzyme with false targets. Co-amoxiclav is useful when the broad spectrum of amoxicillin is required, but β-lactamase-producing organisms, such as *Staph. aureus, H. influenzae, M. catarrhalis, E. coli* or *Bacteroides*, may be involved. It is the first choice for infected animal and human bites. If there is no likelihood of penicillin-resistant infection, use plain amoxicillin instead because it is safer and much cheaper

References

- Medicines and Healthcare Products Regulatory Agency/Committee on Safety of Medicines (1997) *Curr Probl Pharmacovigilance* **23**: 5–8.
- Garcia Rodriguez LA, Stricker BH and Zimmerman HJ (1996) Risk of acute liver injury associated with the combination of amoxicillin and clavulanic acid. *Arch Intern Med* **156**: 1327–33.

[5.1.2] Cefalexin

Class:	cephalosporin β-lactamase-resistant broad-spectrum bactericidal antibacterial
Tablets or capsules:	250, 500 mg
Liquid:	125 mg/5 ml, 250 mg/5 ml
Dose:	adults: 250 mg four times a day, or 500 mg two to three times a day children 6–12 years: 250 mg three times a day 1–5 years: 125 mg three times a day under 1 year: 125 mg twice a day
Pack:	28 (250 mg); 21 (500 mg); 100 ml
$t_{1/2}$:	1 h
Side-effects:	rare, but there may be allergy in people allergic to penicillin (10% cross-over) including rashes, fever and joint pains; diarrhoea and, rarely, antibiotic-associated colitis, especially with high doses; or, with courses longer than 2 weeks, reduced white cells or platelets, liver or kidney damage which should recover once the drug is stopped
Interactions:	warfarin effect may be altered, slight reduction in efficacy of combined oral contraceptive pill
Cautions:	penicillin sensitivity, renal impairment, porphyria. The efficacy of this antibiotic can be impaired by storage at high room temperatures
Selection:	cephalosporins are similar to β-lactamase-resistant penicillins in their action and their clinical use. Cefalexin is useful in treating urinary tract infections in pregnancy where the sensitivity of the infecting organism is not yet known and trimethoprim is not licensed for use

Reference

- Crichton B (2004) Keep in a cool place: exposure of medicines to high temperatures in general practice during a British heatwave. *J R Soc Med* **97**: 328–9.

[5.1.3] Doxycycline (NPEF)

Class:	tetracycline broad-spectrum bacteriostatic anti-bacterial
Capsules or dispersible tablets:	100 mg
Dose:	adults: 200 mg on first day, then 100 mg daily; capsules should be swallowed whole with plenty of fluid during meals, while sitting or standing, and at least 1 h before retiring to bed
Pack:	8
$t_{1/2}$:	16 (12–24) h (probably decreased by alcohol)
Side-effects:	photosensitivity (minimise exposure to strong sunlight or sunlamps), nausea, vomiting, dysphagia and oesophageal irritation (hence the instruction about how to take the medication); diarrhoea and rarely antibiotic-associated colitis; very rarely headache and visual disturbances which may indicate 'benign' intracranial hypertension, also rarely reported cases of hypoglycaemia in non-diabetic people
Interactions:	antacids (also quinapril which contains magnesium carbonate), iron, zinc, oral bismuth chelate (Pepto-Bismol® or De-Nol®), warfarin, antiepileptics, barbiturates, alcohol, rifampicin, slight reduction in efficacy of combined oral contraceptive pill; avoid prescribing with ciclosporin or retinoids; avoid prescribing this bacteriostatic drug with a bactericidal antibiotic such as a penicillin, because the two mechanisms of action interfere with each other
Cautions:	**avoid prescribing in pregnancy**, breastfeeding, hepatic impairment, systemic lupus erythematosus (SLE), porphyria. **Not for children under 12 years of age**
Selection:	doxycycline is well absorbed from the gut and not affected by food, or calcium-rich food which does affect other tetracyclines. It is eliminated via the bile and the faeces as well as in the urine, so there is no need to adjust the dose in mild or moderate renal impairment

References

- Digre KB (2003) Not so benign intracranial hypertension. *BMJ* **326**: 613–14.
- Lochhead J and Elston JS (2003) Doxycycline induced intracranial hypertension. *BMJ* **326**: 641–2.
- Al-Mofarreh MA and Al Mofleh IA (2003) Esophageal ulceration complicating doxycycline therapy. *World J Gastroenterol* **9**: 609–11.

[5.1.5] Erythromycin (NPEF)

Class:	macrolide bacteriostatic antibiotic
Enteric-coated tablets:	250, 500 mg
Liquid:	125 mg/5 ml, 250 mg/5 ml
Dose:	all four times a day, may be doubled for severe infections adults and children 8 years or older: 250 mg (enteric-coated tablets) children (liquid) 2–8 years: 250 mg up to 2 years: 125 mg
Pack:	no specific number of tablets per pack but usual prescription is for 20–28; 100 ml or 140 ml
$t_{1/2}$:	2 h
Side-effects:	nausea or vomiting (20% of patients), abdominal discomfort, diarrhoea (mainly after large doses), antibiotic-associated colitis; allergic reactions; reversible hearing loss also reported after large doses; if given for more than 14 days may occasionally cause cholestatic jaundice
Interactions:	artemether/lumefantrine, atorvastatin, bromocriptine, buspirone, cabergoline, **carbamazepine**, cilostazol, **cimetidine**, clozapine, ciclosporin, digoxin, disopyramide, eletriptan, ergotamine, lercanidipine, loratadine, **mizolastine**, methysergide, **pimozide**, reboxetine, rifabutin, sertindole, sildenafil, **simvastatin**, sirolimus, tacrolimus, tadalafil, **terfenadine**, **theophylline**, tolterodine, valproate, vardenafil, **warfarin**, zopiclone. There is no loss of protection against pregnancy from oral contraceptives
Cautions:	hepatic and severe renal impairment; avoid in porphyria

continued opposite

Selection:

erythromycin binds to ribosomes within bacteria and interferes with protein synthesis. As Gram-positive organisms (e.g. streptococci, staphylococci) absorb the drug more readily, they are more susceptible to its action than Gram-negative ones. The spectrum of activity is similar to penicillin with additional activity against chlamydia and unusual organisms such as mycoplasma and legionella, so it is often used as a substitute when the patient is allergic to penicillin. The only liquid form available is erythromycin ethyl succinate, whereas the generic tablets are erythromycin base in an enteric coating to protect the drug against destruction by gastric acid. Doses for children are set to take into account this difference. There are a number of preparations for adults without any evidence of one being superior to another, but there is a wide range in the prices. Generic enteric-coated tablets are the cheapest

References

- Anonymous (1995) Giving erythromycin by mouth. *Drug Ther Bull* **33**: 77–9.
- Yakatan GJ, Rasmussen CE, Feis PJ and Wallen S (1985) Bioinequivalence of erythromycin ethylsuccinate and enteric-coated erythromycin pellets following multiple oral doses. *J Clin Pharmacol* **25**: 36–42.

[5.1.5] Clarithromycin

Class:	macrolide bacteriostatic antibacterial
Tablets:	250, 500 mg
Liquid:	125 mg/5 ml, 250 mg/5 ml
Granules:	250 mg/sachet
Dose:	all twice a day adults: 250–500 mg children: *see* Table 10.1
Pack:	14 tablets or sachets; 70 ml, 100 ml of 125 mg/5 ml; 70 ml of 250 mg/5 ml
$t_{1/2}$:	3 h after 250 mg; 5 h after 500 mg; but the active metabolite is eliminated slightly slower
Side-effects:	may cause similar side-effects to erythromycin but nausea or vomiting only affect 5% of patients; also dyspepsia, headache, smell and taste disturbances, oral inflammation or discolouration, joint or muscle aches, pancreatitis or hepatitis, various psychological disturbances, renal failure, reduction in white blood cells or platelets
Interactions:	artemether/lumefantrine, atorvastatin, bromocriptine, cabergoline, **carbamazepine**, **cimetidine**, clozapine, ciclosporin, digoxin, disopyramide, eletriptan, ergotamine, itraconazole, methysergide, **mizolastine**, omeprazole, phenytoin, **pimozide**, reboxetine, repaglinide, rifabutin, sertindole, **simvastatin**, sirolimus, tacrolimus, tadalafil, **terfenadine**, **theophylline**, tolterodine, **warfarin**, zopiclone. There is no loss of protection against pregnancy from oral contraceptives
Cautions:	hepatic and renal impairment; pregnancy and breast-feeding; avoid in porphyria
Selection:	this macrolide is an alternative to erythromycin, especially when the patient has experienced nausea with erythromycin. It has a similar spectrum of antimicrobial activity

Reference

• Periti P, Mazzei T, Mini E and Novelli A (1993) Adverse effects of macrolide antibacterials. [Review] *Drug Saf* **9**: 346–64.

Table 10.1 Children's doses of clarithromycin, all twice daily

Weight (kg)	Age (years)	Dose (mg)	Volume of 125 mg/5 ml	Volume of 250 mg/5 ml
30–40	10–12	250	10	5
20–29	7–9	187.5	7.5	–
12–19	3–6	125	5	–
8–11	1–2	62.5	2.5	–
under 8	under 1	7.5 mg/kg	0.3 ml/kg	–

[5.1.8] Trimethoprim (NPEF)

Class:	enzyme-inhibiting bacteriostatic antibacterial
Tablets:	100 mg, 200 mg
Liquid:	50 mg/5 ml
Dose:	all twice a day adults: 200mg children 6–12 years: 100 mg 6 months–5 years: 50 mg 6 weeks–5 months: 25 mg
Pack:	no specific pack size of tablets (usually 6); 100 ml liquid
$t_{1/2}$:	10 h
Side-effects:	blood and generalised skin disorders, especially in the elderly or with long-term treatment; gastro-intestinal disturbances including nausea and vomiting, allergic reactions, raised blood potassium
Interactions:	antimalarial drugs containing pyrimethamine (Fansidar® and Maloprim®), azathioprine, ciclosporin, mercaptopurine, methotrexate, phenytoin, warfarin. Does not affect the combined oral contraceptive pill
Cautions:	breast-feeding, renal impairment, avoid in pregnancy, porphyria, blood disorders
Selection:	trimethoprim inhibits an enzyme (dihydrofolate reductase) which is essential for the metabolism of folic acid. It capitalises on the marked sensitivity of

continued overleaf

the bacterial enzyme relative to the human one. Thus although the antibiotic is not licensed for use in pregnancy and should not be used, many women have taken it before knowing they were pregnant and had no ill-effects. It is a first-line choice for the treatment of uncomplicated urinary infections, but inadequate for more serious ones, such as pyelonephritis. Approximately 10–20% of bacteria responsible for UTI in general practice are resistant to trimethoprim (source via Prodigy). A 3-day course for any age group provides appropriate duration of treatment and patient acceptability, although there is still some controversy that it may have a slightly higher failure rate than a 5-day course

References

- Lutters M and Vogt N (2002) Antibiotic duration for treating uncomplicated, symptomatic lower urinary tract infections in elderly women (Cochrane Review). *The Cochrane Library, Issue 3, 2002*. Update Software, Oxford.
- Michael M, Hodson EM, Craig JC, Martin S and Moyer VA (2003) Short versus standard duration oral antibiotic therapy for acute urinary tract infection in children (Cochrane Review). *The Cochrane Library, Issue 1, 2003*. Update Software, Oxford.
- Goettsch WG, Janknegt R and Hering RMC (2004) Increased treatment failure after 3-days' courses of nitrofurantoin and trimethoprim for urinary tract infections in women: a population-based retrospective cohort study using the PHARMO database. *Br J Clin Pharmacol* **58**: 184–9.

[5.1.11] Metronidazole (NPEF)

Class:	Azole bacteriostatic anti-anaerobic
Tablets:	200, 400 mg
Dose:	200 mg three times a day for seven days for dental infections, 400mg twice a day for seven days *or* 2 g as a single dose for bacterial vaginosis (different dosage regimens are used for other infections)
Pack:	no specific pack size of tablets (usually 20)
$t_{1/2}$:	8 h
Side-effects:	nausea (metallic taste in mouth), vomiting and gastrointestinal disturbances, rashes; rarely drowsiness, headache, dizziness, ataxia, hepatitis, blood disorders, aching, darkening of urine
Interactions:	**alcohol** (interaction may cause facial flushing, throbbing headache, palpitations, nausea and vomiting), **warfarin**, cimetidine, phenytoin, lithium
Cautions:	alcoholism, liver disease
Selection:	metronidazole is the first-line antibiotic used in the UK against anaerobic infections. In the context of treating minor illness, dental infections are quite commonly presented to health professionals other than dentists, and most acute cases of toothache involve infection which can be appropriately treated with amoxicillin and/or metronidazole

Reference

- Palmer NA, Pealing R, Ireland RS and Martin MV (2000) A study of therapeutic antibiotic prescribing in National Health Service general dental practice in England. *Br Dent J* **188**(10): 554–8.

[5.1.13] Nitrofurantoin m/r (NPEF)

Class:	multiple action bactericidal antibacterial
Modified release capsules:	100 mg
Dose:	100 mg twice a day
Pack:	14
$t_{1/2}$:	20 min–1 h, but use of the modified-release version prolongs the action considerably
Side-effects:	urine may be coloured yellow or brown, anorexia, nausea and vomiting (modified release version less so), diarrhoea, acute and chronic pulmonary reactions, peripheral neuropathy; also reported rash, pruritus, hepatitis, pancreatitis, arthralgia, blood disorders and transient alopecia
Interactions:	magnesium trisilicate, probenecid, sulfinpyrazone
Cautions:	avoid in renal failure, late pregnancy, breast-feeding, glucose-6-phosphate dehydrogenase (G6PD) deficiency or porphyria; caution in anaemia, diabetes mellitus, electrolyte imbalance, vitamin B and folate deficiency, hepatic impairment, pulmonary disease, susceptibiliity to peripheral neuropathy
Selection:	approximately 10% of bacteria responsible for UTI in general practice are resistant to nitrofurantoin (source via Prodigy). The antibacterial action of nitrofurantoin is unusual. Nitrofurantoin is converted to an active metabolite that interferes with many essential components of bacterial chemistry. Perhaps this multiple action accounts for the stable level of bacterial resistance, which has not increased appreciably since the antibacterial was first launched in 1953. As it is concentrated in the urine it is highly effective against lower urinary tract infections, but the plasma levels are not sufficient to treat invasive infections such as pyelonephritis. There is less evidence for the use of short 3-day courses for treating uncomplicated lower urinary tract infection with nitrofurantoin than with amoxicillin or trimethoprim, so prescribe a 7-day course. It can be used in pregnancy but not at term because of a risk of neonatal haemolysis

continued opposite

References

- Goettsch WG, Janknegt R and Hering RMC (2004) Increased treatment failure after 3-days' courses of nitrofurantoin and trimethoprim for urinary tract infections in women: a population-based retrospective cohort study using the PHARMO database. *Br J Clin Pharmacol* **58**: 184–9.
- Spencer RC, Moseley DJ and Greensmith MJ (1994) Nitrofurantoin modified release versus trimethoprim or co-trimoxazole in the treatment of uncomplicated urinary tract infection in general practice. *J Antimicrob Chemother* **33** (Suppl A): 121–9.

[5.2] Fluconazole (OTC)

Class:	triazole antifungal
Capsules:	150 mg
Dose:	(vaginal candidiasis) 150 mg single dose
Pack:	1
$t_{1/2}$:	30 h
Side-effects:	occasionally nausea, abdominal discomfort, diarrhoea, flatulence; rarely headache, hepatic disorders, skin reactions, seizures, reduced white cells or platelets, allergic reactions
Interactions:	avoid with eletroptan, pimozide, sertindole, sirolimus, tacrolimus, terfenadine. There are many interactions between triazole antifungal and other drugs, but most, with the exception of those just listed, may be irrelevant to the use of a single dose of the antifungal
Cautions:	avoid in pregnancy and breast-feeding
Selection:	fluconazole is available OTC to people aged 16–60 years for the treatment of vaginal thrush and associated candidal balanitis as a single dose pack of 150 mg. Some women find it more acceptable than using a pessary, but it is no more effective and costs a few pounds more

Reference

- Watson MC, Grimshaw JM, Bond CM, Mollison J and Ludbrook A (2003) Oral versus intra-vaginal imidazole and triazole anti-fungal treatment of uncomplicated vulvo-vaginal candidiasis (thrush) (Cochrane Review). *The Cochrane Library, Issue 1, 2003.* Update Software, Oxford.

[5.2] Nystatin (NPEF)

Class:	polyene antifungal
Liquid:	100 000 units/ml
Dose:	children and infants: 1 ml four times a day
Pack:	30 ml with pipette
$t_{1/2}$:	not absorbed
Side-effects:	oral irritation
Interactions:	none
Cautions:	although it is used, it is not licensed for use in infants aged under 1 month
Selection:	nystatin is not absorbed from the gut, so it is most unlikely to cause any systemic side-effects. It was named after being discovered in New York State, derived from soil fungi actinomycetes. Despite its safety, it is still a prescription-only medicine

[5.5.1] Mebendazole (OTC)

Class:	antihelmintic
Tablets (chewable):	100 mg
Liquid:	100 mg/5 ml
Dose:	for threadworms adults and children aged 2 years and older: 100 mg single dose (if re-infection occurs, a second dose may be needed after 2–3 weeks)
Pack:	6 tablets; 30 ml
$t_{1/2}$:	1 h
Side-effects:	rarely abdominal pain, diarrhoea, headache, dizziness, allergic reactions
Interactions:	cimetidine
Cautions:	avoid in pregnancy (toxicity in rats), no information about safety in breast-feeding
Selection:	this is the first-line treatment for treating threadworm infestations in anyone aged 2 years or over. It is not suitable for use in pregnancy because toxicity has been demonstrated in animal studies. As there is no suitable alternative treatment during early pregnancy, pregnant women may have to put up with threadworms until after the first trimester, but thereafter piperazine can be used

References

- Dawson M, Braithwaite PA, Roberts MS and Watson TR (1985) The pharmacokinetics and bioavailability of a tracer dose of [3H]-mebendazole in man. *Br J Clin Pharmacol* **19**: 79–86.
- www.prodigy.nhs.uk/guidance.asp?gt=threadworm (accessed 13 June 2005)

[5.5.1] Piperazine (OTC)

Class:	antihelmintic
Oral powder:	for mixing into milk or water: piperazine phosphate 4 g, sennosides 15.3 mg per sachet
Dose:	for threadworms two doses are given, two weeks apart adults: 1 sachet at bedtime children aged 2 years or older: use mebendazole 1 year–1 year 11 months: 5ml of sachet contents in the morning 3 months–1 year: 2.5 ml of sachet contents in the morning
Pack:	2 sachets
$t_{1/2}$:	wide variation between individuals, but usually fully eliminated within 24 h
Side-effects:	nausea, vomiting, colic, diarrhoea, allergic reactions, seizures
Interactions:	none
Cautions:	avoid in liver impairment, first trimester of pregnancy (manufacturer's advice), severe renal impairment, or epilepsy; if breast-feeding, express and discard breast milk for 8 h after the dose
Selection:	this is the alternative treatment for threadworm infestations when mebendazole cannot be used

Reference

• Leach FN (1990) Management of threadworm infestation during pregnancy. [Review] *Arch Dis Child* **65**: 399–400.

Endocrine system

[6.4.1.2] Norethisterone (NPEF)

Class:	progestogen
Tablets:	5 mg
Dose:	to delay menstruation: 5 mg three times a day, starting 3 days before expected menstrual period
Pack:	30
$t_{1/2}$:	8 (5–12) h
Side-effects:	fluid retention, weight gain, nausea, change in libido, breast discomfort, headache, dizziness, insomnia, drowsiness, depression, skin reactions including exacerbation of acne, jaundice, allergic reactions
Interactions:	ciclosporin, warfarin, antidiabetic drugs; drugs that accelerate the metabolism of progestogens and reduce the effectiveness of progestogen-only contraceptives could reduce the effectiveness of norethisterone used to delay a period
Cautions:	pregnancy, breast-feeding, arterial disease, susceptibility to thromboembolism, epilepsy, uncontrolled hypertension, cardiac failure, renal or liver impairment, migraine, depression, diabetes
Selection:	norethisterone is useful to delay an inconvenient period. Side-effects are quite common but usually mild, with breast tenderness and fluid retention. Bleeding occurs two to three days after stopping the norethisterone. Women taking a standard combined oral contraceptive pill do not need norethisterone for this purpose; they can simply continue without having a 7-day gap between packs. Norethisterone is a synthetic progestogen related to testosterone. Be aware that there has been some publicity that such progestogens may cause an increased risk of breast cancer, but there is no good evidence for this claim

Reference

- Kuhl H (2000) Scientific comment: norethisterone acetate (NETA) – A risky compound? *Geburtshilfe und Frauenheilkunde* **60**: 393–406.

Obstetrics and gynaecology

[7.2.2] Clotrimazole (OTC)

Class:	imidazole antifungal
External cream:	2%
Pessaries:	500 mg
Vaginal cream:	10%
Dose:	for vaginal thrush: one 500 mg pessary or 5 g of 10% vaginal cream inserted at night
Pack:	20 g external cream; 1 pessary with applicator; combination pack with 1 pessary and 10 g external cream; vaginal cream 5g with applicator
$t_{1/2}$:	not applicable (external)
Side-effects:	possible destructive effect on latex condoms and diaphragms (use alternative contraception for at least 5 days after dose), local irritation; rarely allergic reactions
Interactions:	none
Cautions:	some women develop an allergy to the excipients, which may produce symptoms similar to the original infection
Selection:	The usual treatment for vaginal thrush is a single dose of a 500 mg pessary inserted at night. Some women may prefer to use the 10% vaginal cream. External infection can be treated with 2% cream, but this is not sufficient if there is concurrent vaginal infection. Clotrimazole can be used in pregnancy

Reference

- Watson MC, Grimshaw JM, Bond CM, Mollison J and Ludbrook A (2003) Oral versus intra-vaginal imidazole and triazole anti-fungal treatment of uncomplicated vulvovaginal candidiasis (thrush) (Cochrane Review). *The Cochrane Library, Issue 1, 2003*. Update Software, Oxford.

[7.3.1] Levonorgestrel (OTC to women aged 16 years or over, NPEF)

Class:	post-coital contraceptive
Tablets:	750 µg
Dose:	1.5 mg (2 tablets) as soon as possible after unprotected sexual intercourse: best within 12 h, ideally not later than 72 h, but some effect up to 120 h (unlicensed use)
Pack:	2 tablets
$t_{1/2}$:	10 (9–14.5) h
Side-effects:	nausea (affecting 14–23% of patients), lower abdominal pain (18%), fatigue (17%), headache (17%), dizziness (11%), breast tenderness (11%), vomiting (6%). Glucose tolerance may worsen. The timing of menstrual bleeding may be temporarily disturbed, although most women have their next period on time. If it is more than 1 week overdue, a pregnancy test is needed. A barrier method will need to be used until the next period. Also advise the patient to report any lower abdominal pains, which might indicate an ectopic pregnancy
Interactions:	drugs that induce liver enzymes reduce the effectiveness of the contraception. The drugs suspected of doing this are: carbamazepine, griseofulvin, phenytoin, primodone, rifabutin, rifampicin, ritonavir, St John's Wort. If levonorgestrel is still considered the best option, the dose may need to be increased to 2.25mg (3 tablets). There is also an interaction with ciclosporin which could lead to toxic effects
Cautions:	check that there was no earlier unprotected intercourse during the same cycle that would be outside the time limit. Although hormonal post-coital contraception may work up to 120 h after intercourse, the effectiveness decreases with time, so the alternative of an intra-uterine device may be a better option. Also check that a period is not overdue which may be because the woman is already pregnant. If vomiting

continued overleaf

occurs within 3 h of taking the dose, repeat with domperidone. Severe malabsorption, such as in severe Crohn's disease, could affect the absorption of the drug. Avoid in pregnancy, porphyria or severe liver disease

Selection: levonorgestrel has now superseded other hormonal methods of oral post-coital contraception

References

- Anonymous (1998) Randomised controlled trial of levonorgestrel versus the Yuzpe regimen of combined oral contraceptives for emergency contraception. Task Force on Postovulatory Methods of Fertility Regulation. *Lancet* **352**: 428–33.
- Webb A, Shochet T, Bigrigg A *et al.* (2004) Effect of hormonal emergency contraception on bleeding patterns. *Contraception* **69**: 133–5.
- Sheffer-Mimouni G, Pauzner D, Maslovitch S, Lessing JB and Gamzu R (2003) Ectopic pregnancies following emergency levonorgestrel contraception. *Contraception* **67**: 267–9.

Nutrition and blood

[9.1.1] Ferrous sulphate (OTC)

Class:	iron
Tablets:	200 mg
Dose:	adults only: usual dose 200 mg three times a day
Pack:	no specific number of tablets but usual supply is 84
$t_{1/2}$:	not applicable as iron is used and stored within the body rather than eliminated
Side-effects:	*reduce dose if side-effects occur* – nausea, epigastric pain, constipation (particularly in the elderly) or diarrhoea
Interactions:	reduced absorption of iron with magnesium trisilicate, tetracyclines, and zinc, trientine. Iron reduces absorption of tetracyclines (e.g. doxycycline), quinolone antibiotics including ciprofloxacin, levothyroxine (take iron and levothyroxine at least 2 h apart), L-dopa, entacapone, biphosphonates, penicillamine and zinc
Cautions:	dangerous to children in overdose
Selection:	this is only used for treating iron deficiency, which usually manifests as microcytic anaemia. A low haemoglobin level frequently occurs in pregnancy, due to dilution. If the mean cell volume is normal, iron deficiency is unlikely. Side-effects are related to the dose of iron rather than the formulation. Some other more expensive forms may seem to give rise to fewer side-effects, but this may well be because less iron is available for absorption. Taking the iron with food reduces both the absorption and the chance of side-effects. There is no point in advocating a diet rich in vitamin C to help improve the absorption, because this only works by converting ferric iron in food to the more readily absorbed ferrous form. As ferrous sulphate is already in this form, adding vitamin C gives no advantage

Reference

- Mahomed K (1997) Iron and folate supplementation in pregnancy (Cochrane Review). *The Cochrane Library, Issue 4, 1997.* Update Software, Oxford.

[9.2.1.2] Dioralyte® (OTC)

Class:	oral rehydration
Sachets:	blackcurrant, citrus or plain; mix one sachet with 200 ml drinking water, use within 1 h or keep in fridge for up to 24 h
Dose:	according to fluid loss, but usually adults: 200–400 ml after every loose motion children 2–12 years: 200 ml after every loose motion infants up to 2 years: 1–1.5 times usual feed volume
Pack:	6 or 20
$t_{1/2}$:	not applicable
Side-effects:	potentially electrolyte imbalance could arise if the solution was incorrectly diluted
Interactions:	none
Cautions:	none
Selection:	having experienced the distribution of a recipe by a health authority for a home-made oral rehydration fluid mixture only to see it rapidly withdrawn when it was discovered that the quantity of salt was incorrect, using manufactured sachets containing the correct amount seems a safer option. If professionals can get the mixture wrong, then so can parents. For those who are normally healthy in affluent countries with plentiful drinking water, oral rehydration with electrolyte–water mixtures is rarely necessary; what matters is maintaining adequate fluid intake and restarting feeding as soon as possible. Note that rehydration fluids used in Britain have less salt and more glucose than the World Health Organization formulation

References

- Mecrow IK and Miller V (1993) An open triple crossover study comparing water absorption from potable water, Lucozade, and Dioralyte using the stable isotope ^{18}O. *J Pediatr Gastroenterol Nutr* **16**: 316–20.
- Hahn S, Kim Y and Garner P (2001) Reduced osmolarity oral rehydration solution for treating dehydration due to diarrhoea in children: systematic review. *BMJ* **323**: 81–5.
- Ho TF, Yip WCL, Duggan C and Vashishtha VM (2001) Letters about oral rehydration solutions. *BMJ* **323**: 1068.

Musculoskeletal system

[10.1.1] Ibuprofen (OTC)

Class:	non-steroidal anti-inflammatory drug
Tablets:	200, 400, 600 mg
Liquid:	100 mg/5 ml (*see* next entry for topical gel)
Dose:	all three or four times a day adults: 400–600 mg children 8–12 years: 200 mg (10 ml) 3–7 years: 100 mg (5 ml) 1–2 years: 50 mg (2.5 ml) *equivalent to 20 mg per kg body weight per day,* not recommended for children weighing under 7 kg
Pack:	84 tablets (but only prescribe the amount required); 100 or 150 ml liquid
$t_{1/2}$:	2 h
Side-effects:	gastrointestinal discomfort – also nausea, diarrhoea, and occasionally bleeding and ulceration, hypersensitivity reactions – notably with bronchospasm, rashes and angio-oedema. Other rare side-effects include fluid retention, headache, dizziness, vertigo, changes in mood, hearing disturbances such as tinnitus, photosensitivity, haematuria, blood disorders, renal failure, alveolitis, hepatic damage, pancreatitis, eye changes and aseptic meningitis
Interactions:	ibuprofen co-administered with aspirin can not only increase the risk of gastrointestinal haemorrhage but may also counteract the protective effect of aspirin against thrombosis. Other interactions with: ciclosporin, lithium, methotrexate, penicillamine, pentoxyifylline, phenytoin, quinolones (such as ciprofloxacin), SSRI antidepressants (such as fluoxetine), sulphonylureas (such as gliclazide), tacrolimus, warfarin

continued overleaf

Cautions:	• gastrointestinal disease – especially a history of peptic ulcer
	• asthma: about 5% of adults find that *aspirin* causes or exacerbates wheezing. There is a concern that the same effect may occur with ibuprofen and a few case reports of such, but no broad epidemiological evidence. Furthermore, children have fewer problems with asthma when febrile illnesses are treated with ibuprofen instead of paracetamol. The exacerbation of asthma caused by ibuprofen in individuals who are not specifically allergic to it, may turn out to be as much a myth as the misconception that ibuprofen was ineffective in women
	• allergy to aspirin or other NSAID
	• elderly, pregnancy, heart, kidney or liver disease
	• systemic lupus erythematosus
Selection:	of the group of standard NSAIDs, ibuprofen poses the least risk of gastrointestinal bleeding. Toxicity to the gut is mainly from the systemic effect of ibuprofen, not a local effect, so it makes little difference whether it is taken after food or not

References

• Body R and Potier K (2004) Non-steroidal anti-inflammatory drugs and exacerbations of asthma in children. *Emerg Med J* **21**: 713.
• Khazaeinia T and Jamali F (2000) Evaluation of gastrointestinal toxicity of ibuprofen using surrogate markers in rats: effect of formulation and route of administration. *Clin Exp Rheumatol* **18**: 187–92.
• MacDonald TM and Wei L (2003) Effect of ibuprofen on cardioprotective effect of aspirin. *Lancet* **361**: 57.
• Anonymous (2004) Mythbuster: ibuprofen and women. *Bandolier* **120**: 4.

[10.3.2] Ibuprofen (topical) (OTC)

Class:	non-steroidal anti-inflammatory drug
Gel:	10%
Dose:	apply three times daily
Pack:	30, 100 g
$t_{1/2}$:	although the plasma half-life is 2 h, levels in the blood are very low with topical formulations. Ibuprofen can be detected at therapeutically effective concentration in soft tissue under the area of application for at least 15 h afterwards
Side-effects:	rarely, allergic reactions including asthma and rashes; dyspepsia, exacerbation of renal impairment
Interactions:	most unlikely with topical form
Cautions:	as for oral ibuprofen, but much less likely to pose a significant risk
Selection:	higher concentrations of ibuprofen are found in soft tissue in the area of application using a topical formulation than with an oral form, but there is hardly any penetration into large joints. Therefore the percutaneous route is ideal for soft tissue inflammatory conditions but not suitable for relieving arthritic pains. Gel formulations provide better absorption than emulsions

References

- Dominkus M, Nicolakis M, Kotz R et al. (1996) Comparison of tissue and plasma levels of ibuprofen after oral and topical administration. *Arzneimittel-Forschung* **46**: 1138–43.
- Treffel P and Gabard B (1993) Ibuprofen epidermal levels after topical application in vitro: effect of formulation, application time, dose variation and occlusion. *Br J Dermatol* **129**: 286–91.
- Vaile JH and Davis P (1998) Topical NSAIDs for musculoskeletal conditions. A review of the literature. [Review] *Drugs* **56**: 783–99.

[10.3.2] Algesal® (OTC)

Class:	counter-irritant
Cream:	diethylamine salicylate 10%
Dose:	adults and children 6 years or over: massage in three times a day, wash hands afterwards
Pack:	50 g
$t_{1/2}$:	not applicable
Side-effects:	local irritation
Interactions:	none
Cautions:	none
Selection:	counter-irritants relieve pain by causing sensation from the skin to block the entry of pain stimuli into the spinal cord via the same nerve. They are simple to use because even if the pain is referred, the best place to apply the cream is where the pain is felt. There is little evidence to choose between the wide variety of preparations available, and Algesal is inexpensive

Reference

- Mason L, Moore RA, Edwards JE *et al.* (2004) Systematic review of efficacy of topical rubefacients containing salicylates for the treatment of acute and chronic pain [see comment]. [Review] *BMJ* **328**: 995.

Eye

[11.3.1] Chloramphenicol (OTC drops for adults and children 2 years and over, NPEF)

Class:	topical, primarily bacteriostatic, antibiotic
Drops:	0.5%
Ointment:	1%
Dose:	drops: apply hourly at first, reduce to 4-hourly as symptoms improve; ointment: apply four times a day, or at night if used in conjunction with drops
Pack:	10 ml drops or 4 g ointment
$t_{1/2}$:	5 h – but not relevant to topical use because so little is absorbed
Side-effects:	transient stinging
Interactions:	none
Cautions:	past or close family history of blood disorder
Selection:	chloramphenicol has a broad spectrum of activity, but its systemic use is limited by rare but serious toxicity. Topical use is free from this hazard. The risk of serious blood disorders among people who have used topical chloramphenicol is no higher than the background rate, but the reassurance gained from this does not necessarily apply to patients who have a past or close family history of such disorders, who could be more susceptible. The patient information leaflet warns of this

Reference

- Laporte JR, Vidal X, Ballarin E and Ibanez L (1998) Possible association between ocular chloramphenicol and aplastic anaemia – the absolute risk is very low. *Br J Clin Pharmacol* **46**: 181–4.

[11.4.2] Sodium cromoglicate eye drops (OTC)

Class:	preventative anti-inflammatory
Eye drops:	2%
Dose:	adults and children: 1 drop four times a day
Pack:	13.5 ml
$t_{1/2}$:	not applicable to local effect
Side-effects:	transient stinging
Interactions:	none
Cautions:	discard 1 month after opening
Selection:	the mechanism of action of sodium cromoglicate is not as straightforward as simply inhibiting the release of histamine from stores in mast cells. Doubts were cast on this theory many years ago when a study showed beneficial effects on acute asthma, when the drug ought to have none. Nevertheless, the maximum benefit from using this drug is only likely to be gained if it is used regularly throughout the allergic season

References

- Sadeghi-Hashjin G, Nijkamp FP, Henricks PA and Folkerts G (2002) Sodium cromoglycate and doxantrazole are oxygen radical scavengers. *Eur Resp J* **20**: 867–72.
- Anderson SD, Du Toit JI, Rodwell LT and Jenkins CR (1994) Acute effect of sodium cromoglycate on airway narrowing induced by 4.5 percent saline aerosol: Outcome before and during treatment with aerosol corticosteroids in patients with asthma. *Chest* **105**: 673–80.

[11.8.1] Hypromellose (OTC)

Class:	tear replacement
Eye drops:	0.3%
Dose:	use as needed, usually 2 drops three times a day
Pack:	10 ml
$t_{1/2}$:	not applicable
Side-effects:	none
Interactions:	none
Cautions:	discard 1 month after opening
Selection:	hypromellose is the standard solution used to replace deficient tears. Such medication does help the condition but fails to restore the correct composition of the conjunctival mucus. If the patient does not obtain adequate relief with this preparation it is often worth trying an alternative listed in this section of the *BNF*

Reference

• Versura P, Maltarello MC, Stecher F, Caramazza R and Laschi R (1989) Dry eye before and after therapy with hydroxypropyl methylcellulose. Ultrastructural and cytochemical study in 20 patients. *Ophthalmologica* **198**: 152–62.

Ear, nose and oropharynx

[12.1.1] EarCalm® (OTC)

Class:	antibacterial and antifungal topical solution
Spray:	acetic acid 2%
Dose:	adults and children 12 years or over: 1 spray into affected ear(s) three times a day for up to 1 week
Pack:	5 ml
$t_{1/2}$:	not applicable
Side-effects:	transient stinging
Interactions:	none
Cautions:	manufacturer advises treatment for children under 12 years only on medical advice
Selection:	Prodigy describes this treatment for otitis externa as 'a "best guess" treatment for use while awaiting the results of swabs'. As this preparation is available OTC, many people successfully treat themselves for this condition on the advice of their pharmacist, without any need for swabs to be taken. The advantage of simple acetic acid is that it is an antiseptic with a wide range of mild activity against both bacteria and fungi, but without the risk of either sensitisation to an antibiotic, or fungal superinfection caused by topical steroids. The disadvantage of this preparation is that it is not as effective as a corticosteroid plus either acetic acid or antibacterial. There is no steroid/acetic acid preparation marketed in the UK without an antibiotic, so that option is currently unavailable. For more inflamed cases of otitis externa, a topical steroid/antibacterial combination and/or oral antibiotic is recommended

References

- Rowlands S, Devalia H, Smith C, Hubbard R and Dean A (2001) Otitis externa in UK general practice: a survey using the UK General Practice Research Database. *Br J Gen Pract* **51**: 533–8.
- van Balen FA, Smit WM, Zuithoff NP and Verheij TJ (2003) Clinical efficacy of three common treatments in acute otitis externa in primary care: randomised controlled trial. *BMJ* **327**: 1201–5.

[12.1.1] Otosporin®

Class:	bactericidal antibiotics and corticosteroid topical solution
Ear drops:	hydrocortisone 1%, neomycin 3400 units/ml, poly-myxin B 10 000 units/ml
Dose:	3 drops into the ear three times a day
Pack:	5, 10 ml
$t_{1/2}$:	not applicable
Side-effects:	occasional sensitivity reactions, with an increased risk in patients with chronic otitis externa or venous disease such as varicose eczema or ulceration. The drops may sting on application
Interactions:	none
Cautions:	if previous perforation, consult doctor. Avoid prolonged use: usually one week is sufficient. If the condition fails to respond or gets worse, take a swab to identify infections not affected by the antibiotics in Otosporin, such as fungal, but also stop the Otosporin in case the patient has developed a sensitivity to it. Advise the patient not to wash the ear canal using soap or shampoo, as this could inactivate the antibiotics as well as exacerbating the underlying eczema
Selection:	the two antibiotics in this preparation are active against a wide range of bacteria, including *Pseudomonas*. Swabs from infected cases of otitis externa in primary care frequently grow this organism. The fact that patients present more often in the summer months with *Pseudomonas* infection after swimming in pools, suggests that this micro-organism is more than a bystander

References

- Hajjartabar M (2004) Poor-quality water in swimming pools associated with a substantial risk of otitis externa due to *Pseudomonas aeruginosa*. *Water Sci Technol* **50**: 63–7.
- also *see* references above for EarCalm®

[12.1.1] Otomize® (NPEF)

Class:	mixed antibacterials and corticosteroid topical solution
Spray:	dexamethasone 0.1%, neomycin 3250 units/ml, glacial acetic acid 2%
Dose:	1 metered spray drops into the ear three times a day
Pack:	5 ml
$t_{1/2}$:	not applicable
Side-effects:	occasional sensitivity reactions, with an increased risk in patients with chronic otitis externa or eczema. The drops may sting on application
Interactions:	none
Cautions:	if previous perforation, consult doctor. Avoid prolonged use: usually one week is sufficient. If the condition fails to respond or gets worse, take a swab to identify infections not affected by the antibacterials in Otomize, such as fungal, but also stop the Otomize in case the patient has developed a sensitivity to it. Advise the patient not to wash the ear canal using soap or shampoo, as this could inactivate the antibacterials as well as exacerbating the underlying eczema
Selection:	this is a compromise between EarCalm, which depends on acetic acid for its antibacterial action, and Otosporin, which we recommend for infections occurring after swimming. The spray delivery system provides a more accurate dose than self-administered drops, may be more effective and is often preferred by patients

References

- Lancaster J, Mathews J, Williams RS, Thussey C and Kent SE (2003) Comparison of compliance between topical aural medications. *Clin Otolaryngol* **28**: 331–4.
- Connolly AA, Picozzi GL and Browning GG (1997) Randomized trial of neomycin/dexamethasone spray vs drop preparation for the treatment of active chronic mucosal otitis media. *Clin Otolaryngol* **22**: 529–31.
- also *see* references above for EarCalm®

[12.2.1] Beclometasone aqueous nasal spray (OTC)

Class: corticosteroid

Nasal spray: beclometasone 50 µg per spray

Dose: adults and children over 6 years: initially two sprays to each nostril twice daily; when symptoms are controlled reduce to one spray twice daily

Pack: 200-spray unit

$t_{1/2}$:   irrelevant to the local action, but for the small amount absorbed 0.5 h for beclometasone and 2.7 h for its active metabolite

Side-effects: dry nose or throat, epistaxis, altered smell or taste; rarely ulceration of the nasal septum, broncho-spasm, headache, raised intra-ocular pressure or glaucoma, growth retardation in children, allergic reactions

Interactions: none

Cautions: untreated nasal infection, recent nasal surgery, pul-monary tuberculosis, in children on long-term treatment monitor height annually

Selection: with no evidence to suggest superiority of any particular topical steroid for hay fever, the selection is made on the basis of cost. Beclometasone does give benefit on the first day of use, but this increases over the next few days, so ideally patients should start treatment one week before their hay fever season starts. Systemic side-effects are extremely rare because the dose of corticosteroid is so low, nasal absorption is less than 1% and swallowed beclometasone is rapidly cleared

References

- Graft D, Aaronson D, Chervinsky P *et al.* (1996) A placebo- and active-controlled randomized trial of prophylactic treatment of seasonal allergic rhinitis with mometasone furoate aqueous nasal spray. *J Allerg Clin Immunol* **98**: 724–31.
- Selner JC, Weber RW, Richmond GW, Stricker WE and Norton JD (1995) Onset of action of aqueous beclomethasone dipropionate nasal spray in seasonal allergic rhinitis. *Clin Ther* **17**: 1099–109.

[12.2.2] Saline nose drops (OTC)

Class:	topical nasal decongestant
Drops:	sodium chloride 0.9%
Dose:	apply to nostrils before feeds
Pack:	10 ml
$t_{1/2}$:	not applicable
Side-effects:	none
Interactions:	none
Cautions:	none
Selection:	helps to liquefy nasal mucous secretions

Reference

• www.patient.co.uk/showdoc/23069191/ (accessed 13 June 2005)

[12.2.2] Warm moist air inhalation (OTC)

Class:	topical nasal decongestant
Liquid:	very hot water
Dose:	inhale three or four times a day with a towel over the head
Pack:	not applicable
$t_{1/2}$:	not applicable
Side-effects:	only the risk of scalds from the hot water
Interactions:	none
Cautions:	none
Selection:	helps to liquefy nasal mucous secretions. Adding aromatic oils may make the experience more soothing

Reference

• www.patient.co.uk/showdoc/23068821/ (accessed 13 June 2005)

[12.3.4] Chlorhexidine oral spray (OTC)

Class:	antiseptic
Spray:	chlorhexidine gluconate 0.2%
Dose:	up to 12 actuations applied to ulcer(s) twice daily
Pack:	60 ml
$t_{1/2}$:	not applicable
Side-effects:	chlorhexidine has been associated with bitter taste, brown staining of teeth and tongue, and nausea, but these effects are less likely with the limited amount required to cover an oral ulcer with the spray compared with a mouthwash
Interactions:	none
Cautions:	none
Selection:	superficial infection may play a part in the symptoms caused by aphthous ulcers. Chlorhexidine is a general antiseptic with limited evidence of effectiveness in reducing the severity, duration and incidence of oral ulceration

References

- Aphthous ulcers: chlorhexidine and similar agents (2004) *Clinical Evidence* BMJ Publishing Group, London. www.clinicalevidence.com/ceweb/conditions/orh/1303/1303_I2.jsp (accessed 13 June 2005)
- Addy M, Carpenter R and Roberts WR (1976) Management of recurrent aphthous ulceration. A trial of chlorhexidine gluconate gel. *Br Dent J* **141**: 118–20.

Skin

[13.2.1] Emulsifying ointment; hydrous ointment; Oilatum® bath additive (OTC)

Class:	emollients
Dose:	apply in the direction of hair growth as frequently as necessary, or add 1 to 3 capfuls to bath
Pack:	100, 500 g ointments; 250, 500 ml bath additive
$t_{1/2}$:	not applicable
Side-effects:	rarely sensitisation to an excipient in an emollient (consult the listed excipients in the *BNF* or table in *MIMS* to help in choosing an alternative); can make the surface of a bath slippery
Interactions:	none
Cautions:	none
Selection:	emollients hydrate the skin and are useful in all dry or scaling disorders. The choice is mainly a matter of patient preference. Emulsifying ointment can also be used instead of soap

Reference

• Berth-Jones J and Graham-Brown RAC (1992) How useful are soap substitutes? *J Dermatol Treat* **3**: 9–11.

[13.4] Hydrocortisone cream or ointment – *mild* (OTC); Clobetasone butyrate cream or ointment – *moderately potent* (NPEF); betamethasone valerate cream or ointment – *potent* (NPEF)

Class:	topical corticosteroids
Cream or ointment:	hydrocortisone 0.5% or 1%; clobetasone butyrate 0.05%; betamethasone valerate 0.025%, 0.1%
Pack:	hydrocortisone 15, 30 g; clobetasone 30, 100 g; betamethasone 0.025% 100 g; betamethasone 0.1% 30, 100 g
$t_{1/2}$:	not applicable
Side-effects:	worsening of infection including acne, thinning and potential permanent disfiguring marks of skin with potency greater than hydrocortisone, increased hair growth, perioral dermatitis (papular rash around the mouth in young women), depigmentation; large doses may be absorbed into the body and cause similar side-effects to oral steroids; rarely sensitisation to an excipient (consult the listed excipients in the *BNF* or table in *MIMS* to help in choosing an alternative)
Interactions:	none
Cautions:	skin infection including acne, do not use clobetasone or betamethasone on the face, children are more susceptible to side-effects, psoriasis (may rebound or relapse on stopping betamethasone), avoid confusing plain hydrocortisone with hydrocortisone butyrate, or clobetasone with clobetasol, because either switch would inadvertently increase the potency
Selection:	topical corticosteroids are helpful in treating dry skin conditions. The general rule is to use none if an emollient will suffice, otherwise to use the mildest effective potency. Some of the therapeutic effect of these preparations is due to the emollient vehicle

continued overleaf

rather than just the steroid component. Sensitisation to one of the excipients can occur and lead to diagnositic confusion when a dermatitis persists or worsens despite treatment

References

- National Prescribing Centre (1999) Using topical corticosteroids in general practice. *MeReC Bull* **10**: 21–4.
- Anonymous (2003) Topical steroids for atopic dermatitis in primary care. *Drug Ther Bull* **41**: 5–8.
- Parneix-Spake A, Goustas P and Green R (2001) Eumovate (clobetasone butyrate) 0.05% cream with its moisturizing emollient base has better healing properties than hydrocortisone 1% cream: a study in nickel-induced contact dermatitis. *J Dermatol Treat* **12**: 191–7.
- Charman CR, Morris AD and Williams HC (2000) Topical corticosteroid phobia in patients with atopic eczema. *Br J Dermatol* **142**: 931–6.

[13.4] Clotrimazole/hydrocortisone cream (OTC)

Class:	topical antifungal and corticosteroid
Cream or ointment:	clotrimazole 1% and hydrocortisone 1%
Dose:	apply twice daily
Pack:	30 g
$t_{1/2}$:	not applicable
Side-effects:	*see* hydrocortisone
Interactions:	none
Cautions:	*see* hydrocortisone
Selection:	for simple fungal skin infections, use plain clotrimazole topically (*see* section 13.10.2). If pruritus is troublesome, or the fungal infection is in an eczematous area, the combination of an antifungal agent with a corticosteroid can be helpful. Both clotrimazole and miconazole are the same type of imidazole antifungal agents, so if a fungal infection does not respond to one it will not respond to the other. Terbinafine cream is then a suitable alternative

Reference

- Crawford F, Hart R, Bell-Syer S *et al.* (1999) Topical treatments for fungal infections of the skin and nails of the foot (Cochrane Review). *The Cochrane Library, Issue 3, 1999.* Update Software, Oxford.

[13.7] Salicylic acid (OTC)

Class: topical treatment for warts
                 various formulations available from 11% to 26%;
                 currently the least expensive is Salactol®

Dose: apply daily

Pack: 10 ml

$t_{1/2}$:   not applicable

Side-effects: local irritation, sensitisation

Interactions: none

Cautions: flammable

Selection: The limited evidence that is available on the topical
                 treatment of warts suggests salicylic acid is the best

Reference

- Gibbs S, Harvey I, Sterling JC and Stark R (2003) Local treatments for cutaneous warts (Cochrane Review). *The Cochrane Library, Issue 3, 2003*. Update Software, Oxford.

[13.10.1] Sodium fusidate ointment (NPEF)

Class: anti-staphylococcal topical antibiotic

Ointment: 2%

Dose: apply three to four times a day

Pack: 15, 30 g

$t_{1/2}$:   not applicable to local effect

Side-effects: rarely local hypersensitivity reactions

Interactions: none

Cautions: avoid contact with eyes

Selection: this narrow-spectrum antibiotic is very effective against staphylococcal infections. The Cochrane Review of treatment for impetigo concluded that this topical agent is better than oral antibiotics for people with limited disease, and possibly even for those with more extensive disease. We know of no comparative study between fusidic acid cream and sodium fusidate ointment, but it seems more appropriate to use the salt than the acid on areas of skin that are likely to be inflamed and sore. The ointment can also be used to treat angular cheilitis (inflammation of the corners of the lips, which become cracked and sore)

Reference

- Koning S, Verhagen AP, van Suijlekom-Smit LWA *et al.* (2003) Interventions for impetigo (Cochrane Review). *The Cochrane Library, Issue 2, 2003*. Update Software, Oxford.

[13.10.2] Clotrimazole cream (OTC)

Class:	topical antifungal
Cream:	clotrimazole 1%
Dose:	apply twice daily
Pack:	20, 50 g
$t_{1/2}$:	not applicable
Side-effects:	rarely local irritation
Interactions:	may cause damage to latex contraceptives
Cautions:	none
Selection:	for simple fungal skin infections, use plain clotrimazole topically. If pruritis is troublesome, or the fungal infection is in an eczematous area, the combination of an antifungal agent with a corticosteroid can be helpful (*see* section 13.4). Both clotrimazole and miconazole are the same type of imidazole antifungal agents, so if a fungal infection does not respond to one it will not respond to the other. Terbinafine cream is then a suitable alternative

Reference

• Crawford F, Hart R, Bell-Syer S *et al.* (1999) Topical treatments for fungal infections of the skin and nails of the foot (Cochrane Review). *The Cochrane Library, Issue 3, 1999*. Update Software, Oxford.

[13.10.2] Terbinafine cream (OTC)

Class:	allylamine topical antifungal
Cream:	1%
Dose:	apply one to two times a day, for 1 week for fungal infections of the feet, 2 weeks if elsewhere
Pack:	15, 30 g
$t_{1/2}$:	not applicable to local effect
Side-effects:	redness, itching or stinging occasionally occur at the site of application; however, treatment rarely has to be discontinued for this reason. This must be distinguished from allergic reactions which are rare but require discontinuation
Interactions:	none
Cautions:	avoid contact with eyes
Selection:	this broad-spectrum antifungal agent is a useful alternative to clotrimazole because cross-resistance is unusual. Terbinafine can be applied less often and for a shorter course, but is more expensive. The Cochrane Review concluded: 'The most cost-effective strategy is first to treat with azoles or undecenoic acid and to use allylamines only if that fails'

Reference

• Crawford F, Hart R, Bell-Syer S *et al.* (1999) Topical treatments for fungal infections of the skin and nails of the foot (Cochrane Review). *The Cochrane Library, Issue 3, 1999*. Update Software, Oxford.

[13.10.3] Aciclovir cream (OTC)

Class:	topical antiviral
Cream:	aciclovir 5%
Dose:	apply every 4 h (five times a day) for 5 days at the first sign of an attack, continuing for a further 5 days if the lesions have not completely healed
Pack:	2 g
$t_{1/2}$:	not applicable to local effect
Side-effects:	transient stinging or burning; occasionally erythema or drying of the skin, sensitivity to excipients
Interactions:	none (interactions listed in the *BNF* apply to tablets and infusions, not the cream)
Cautions:	avoid contact with eyes and mucous membranes, limited data in pregnancy and breast-feeding – but not known to be harmful
Selection:	aciclovir interferes with viral DNA synthesis. It is used topically to treat cold sores. Standard advice is that the cream needs to be applied as soon as the first symptom appears, and although this gives the best chance of speedy resolution, the cream is still effective if it is applied later. Prophylaxis with topical agents is not effective

References

- Spruance SL and Kriesel JD (2002) Treatment of herpes simplex labialis. [Review] *Herpes* **9**: 64–9.
- Spruance SL, Nett R, Marbury T *et al.* (2002) Acyclovir cream for treatment of herpes simplex labialis: results of two randomized, double-blind, vehicle-controlled, multicenter clinical trials. *Antimicrob Agents Chemother* **46**: 2238–43.

[13.10.4] Malathion (OTC)

Class:	organophosphorus parasiticidal
Liquid:	aqueous malathion 0.5%
Dose:	adults and children over 6 months

head lice: apply liberally to dry hair and scalp, allow to dry naturally, shampoo in the usual way after 12 h, or the next day if preferred, comb the hair, ideally with a fine-toothed metal comb; can be repeated after 7 days (unlicensed use)

scabies: apply over the whole skin surface, do not wash hands after treatment (if any part is washed then reapply malathion to the area afterwards), wash off after 24 h, can be repeated after 7 days (unlicensed use)

Pack:	50, 200 ml (prescribe sufficient to treat the household in case of scabies: children 50 ml, adults 100 ml each)
$t_{1/2}$:	not applicable
Side-effects:	rarely skin irritation
Interactions:	none
Cautions:	avoid contact with eyes, broken or infected skin. Avoid repeated doses at intervals less than one week or for more than three consecutive weeks
Selection:	this is one option to try to tackle the perennial problem of head lice. Scabies is also common. Advise the patient that the irritation from scabies usually lasts for one week after treatment, sometimes up to four weeks, and that it does not represent treatment failure. Malathion is one of the least toxic organophosphorus insecticides because it is rapidly inactived by an enzyme in human plasma

Reference

• Dodd CS (2001) Interventions for treating headlice (Cochrane Review). *The Cochrane Library, Issue 2, 2001*. Update Software, Oxford.

[13.10.4] Permethrin (OTC)

Class:	membrane-destabilising parasiticidal
Cream:	permethrin 5%
Dose:	adults and children over 2 months; scabies: apply over the whole skin surface, do not wash hands after treatment (if any part is washed then reapply permethrin to the area afterwards), wash off after 8–12 h, can be repeated after 7 days
Pack:	30 g (prescribe sufficient to treat the household: children and smaller adults, 30 g larger adults may require two 30 g tubes, the maximum dose for any individual)
$t_{1/2}$:	not applicable
Side-effects:	itching, redness, stinging; rarely rashes, oedema. Permethrin appears to be more toxic to humans than malathion. There are reports of five cases of convulsions and six deaths associated with the topical use of permethrin worldwide, in comparison with two cases of convulsions and no death associated with malathion
Interactions:	none
Cautions:	avoid contact with eyes, broken or infected skin. Ensure you prescribe the 5% strength, not the 1% creme rinse preparation which is intended for head lice but marked as 'less suitable for prescribing' in the *BNF*. Children between 2 months and 2 years should be treated under medical supervision
Selection:	this is an alternative, effective treatment for scabies, but because of the reports of very rare but serious toxicity, malathion would be our first choice. Prodigy recommends permethrin despite the increased risks compared with malathion. Although permethrin would also kill head lice there is no suitable formulation for this use. Only about 0.5% of the applied permethrin is absorbed and that is rapidly metabolised

References

- Walker GJA and Johnstone PW (2000) Interventions for treating scabies (Cochrane Review). *The Cochrane Library, Issue 3, 2000.* Update Software, Oxford.
- WHO (1998) Reported adverse reactions to ectoparasiticodes, incl. scabicides, insecticides and repellants. Abstracted from: WHO Collaborating Centre for International Drug Monitoring, Uppsala, Sweden.

Ideas page

In our experience in managing minor illness, and from talking to other doctors and nurses working in primary care, we have encountered several treatments that appear to be both logical and effective. In the course of researching this book we have sought in vain for any evidence to support these treatments. We list them here to highlight the need for more evidence in these areas, and to invite readers' comments on their own experience of using them.

Boils

- The use of magnesium sulphate paste to 'draw' the purulent material from a boil

Ingrowing toenails

- Teaching the patient to flick the corner of the nail away from the flesh daily, after soaking in water

Pruritus

- Sodium bicarbonate added to the bath
- 2% menthol in aqueous cream

Insect bites

- Witch hazel and piezo-electric devices (such as Zanza-Click)

Burns

- Silver sulphadiazine cream to reduce pain and prevent infection

Haemorrhoids

- Rectal cones (prescribable on FP10) for daily dilation of the anal canal until the condition resolves

Balanitis

- Antibiotics such as fusidic acid in an eye-drop form, to penetrate underneath the foreskin without leaving a sticky residue

Please contact us if you:

- have personal experience of using these treatments
- know of any good research in these areas
- would like to suggest other unproven treatments
- disagree with any of our recommendations, and have evidence to support that view.

Contact options:

Post: Stopsley Group Practice
             Wigmore Lane Health Centre
             Luton, Beds LU2 8BG, UK.
             (This address is due to change in 2006 – please check the website)

Fax: +44 (0)844 884 0138
Website: www.minorillness.co.uk

Useful resources

For the nurse

Books

Essential reference books

- *British National Formulary (BNF)* – updated every 6 months and published by the BMA and Royal Pharmaceutical Society of Great Britain. Make sure you are not using an out-of-date copy! Also available online at www.bnf.org (accessed 13 June 2005).

- *OTC Directory* – published annually by the Proprietary Society of Great Britain. Details (and pictures) of many common over-the-counter preparations.

Other reading

- Ankrett V and Williams I (1999) *Quick Reference Atlas of Dermatology.* MSL.

- Edwards C and Stillman E (2000) *Minor Illness or Major Disease?* Pharmaceutical Press, London.

- Epstein O (2003) *Clinical Examination.* Mosby, London.

- Fry J and Sandler G (1993) *Common Diseases: their nature, prevalence and care.* Petroc Press, Newbury.

- Guillebaud J (2003) *Contraception, Your Questions Answered.* Churchill Livingstone, London.

- Neal MJ (2002) *Medical Pharmacology at a Glance.* Blackwell Science, Oxford.

- Trounce J and Gould D (1999) *Clinical Pharmacology for Nurses.* Churchill Livingstone, London.

Phone

- FPA helpline for contraceptive advice: +44 (0)845 310 1334 (9.00 to 18.00 Monday to Friday).

Online resources

- www.prodigy.co.uk (accessed 13 June 2005): the most useful site for detailed, evidence-based advice on minor illness and reliable patient information sheets

- www.patient.co.uk (accessed 13 June 2005): another useful source of patient information leaflets and self-help groups

- www.library.nhs.uk (accessed 13 June 2005): many useful resources, including the *BNF* and the Cochrane Library

- www.clinicalanswers.nhs.uk (accessed 13 June 2005): A pilot question-answering site set up by the National Library for Health, which will look for evidence to answer your query

- www.peakflow.com (accessed 13 June 2005): for information on the new peak flow meters

- www.dermnetnz.org (accessed 13 June 2005): for skin conditions

- http://emc.medicines.org.uk (accessed 13 June 2005): data sheets (summaries of product characteristics) for all licensed medicines

- www.hpa.org.uk (accessed 13 June 2005): for information on infectiousness

- www.immunisation.nhs.uk (accessed 13 June 2005): current immunisation schedules

- www.dh.gov.uk/PolicyAndGuidance/HealthAndSocialCareTopics/Green Book (accessed 13 June 2005): new chapters of the 'Green Book' *Immunisation Against Infectious Disease* (original version 1996, many new chapters available online)

- www.dh.gov.uk/PolicyAndGuidance/HealthAdviceForTravellers/fs/en (accessed 13 June 2005): for advice about travel

- www.travax.scot.nhs.uk (accessed 13 June 2005): for up-to-date advice about travel vaccination and malaria

- www.dwp.gov.uk/medical/faq.asp (accessed 13 June 2005): for information on sickness certification

DVD

- Davies F (2004) *Spotting the Sick Child*. Department of Health, London (free from 08701 555455 or dh@prolog.uk.com; Stock Number 40630).

For the patient

Reading

- Bishop P (2004) *Relax ... Using Your Own Innate Resources to Let Go of Pent-up Stress and Negative Emotion* (CD-ROM audiobook). HG Publishing, Chalvington (may be hard to obtain in shops: £10 plus £2.50 delivery from +44 (0)1323 811662 or www.humangivens.com (accessed 13 June 2005)).

- Bradley D (2001) *Self-Help for Hyperventilation Syndrome: recognizing and correcting your breathing-pattern disorder.* Hunter House, Alameda, CA.

- Griffin J and Tyrell I (2004) *How to Lift Depression Fast.* HG Publishing, Chalvington.

- Harrold G (2005) *Glenn Harrold's Ultimate Guide to Relaxing Sleep Every Night.* BBC Audiobooks, London.

- Harvey S and Wylie I (1999) *Patient Power: getting the best from your healthcare.* Simon & Schuster, London.

- Servan-Schreiber D (2004) *Healing Without Freud or Prozac: natural approaches to conquering stress, anxiety, depression without drugs and without psychotherapy.* Rodale, London.

- Skynner R and Cleese J (1993) *Families and How to Survive Them.* Vermilion, London.

- Trickett S (1992) *Coping Successfully with Panic Attacks.* Sheldon Press, London.

- Weekes C (2000) *Self-help for Your Nerves: learn to relax and enjoy life again by overcoming stress and fear.* HarperCollins, New York.

Phone

- Samaritans: +44 (0)8457 909090

- Relate: +44 (0)845 130 4010

- National Debtline: +44 (0)808 808 40000

- Consumer Credit Counselling Service: +44 (0)800 138 1111 or www.cccs.co.uk (accessed 13 June 2005)

Abbreviations

AfC	Agenda for Change
BASH	British Association for the Study of Headache
BNF	British National Formulary
BMA	British Medical Association
BP	blood pressure
BTS	British Thoracic Society
CATS	Credit Accumulation and Transfer Scheme
CCDC	Consultant in Communicable Disease Control
COC	combined oral contraceptive
COPD	chronic obstructive pulmonary disease
CSM	Committee on Safety of Medicines
EC	emergency contraception
EFNP	extended formulary nurse prescriber
ESR	erythrocyte sedimentation rate
FBC	full blood count
FPA	Family Planning Association
GMS	General Medical Service
G6PD	glucose-6-phosphate dehydrogenase
GP	general practitioner
HPA	Health Protection Agency
HRT	hormone replacement therapy
5-HT	5-hydroxytryptamine
HVS	high vaginal swab
IV	intravenous
IUCD	intrauterine contraceptive device
LABA	long-acting beta-agonist
LMP	last menstrual period
MAOI	monoamine oxidase inhibitor
MMR	measles, mumps and rubella (vaccination)
m/r	modified release
MRSA	methicillin-resistant *Staphylococcus aureus*
MSU	mid-stream urine
NICE	National Institute for Clinical Excellence
NMC	Nursing and Midwifery Council
NPEF	Nurse Prescribers' Extended Formulary
NSAID	non-steroidal anti-inflammatory drug
OTC	over-the-counter
PCT	primary care trust
PEF	peak expiratory flow

PGD	Patient Group Directions
PHLS	Public Health Laboratory Service
POM	prescription only medicine
RCN	Royal College of Nursing
SLE	systemic lupus erythematosus
SPC	summary of product characteristics
SSRI	selective serotonin reuptake inhibitor
UPSI	unprotected sexual intercourse
UTI	urinary tract infection

Index